T0092123

The Doctor and the Algorithm

Promise, Peril, and the Future of Health AI

S. SCOTT GRAHAM

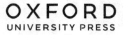

OXFORD
UNIVERSITY PRESS

Oxford University Press is a department of the University of Oxford. It furthers
the University's objective of excellence in research, scholarship, and education
by publishing worldwide. Oxford is a registered trade mark of Oxford University
Press in the UK and certain other countries.

Published in the United States of America by Oxford University Press
198 Madison Avenue, New York, NY 10016, United States of America.

Library of Congress Control Number: 2022908882

ISBN 978-0-19-764446-1

DOI: 10.1093/oso/9780197644461.001.0001

9 8 7 6 5 4 3 2 1

Printed by Sheridan Books, Inc., United States of America

CONTENTS

ACKNOWLEDGMENTS

One of my main goals for *The Doctor and the Algorithm* was to bring together scholarship in critical algorithm studies and AI-focused bioethics research. This simply would not have been feasible without the work of many excellent scholars who have already done so much in these areas. Therefore, many of the most important acknowledgments for this book can be found in my works cited. Additionally, I would like to take this opportunity to thank my friends and colleagues who were generous enough to discuss emerging ideas with me and/or read early drafts of selected chapters: Joshua Barbour, Zoltan Majdik, Justin Rousseau, Casey Boyle, Christa Teston, Caroline Gottschalk-Druschke, and Jodi Nicotra. I also offer sincere thanks to Sarah Humphreville of Oxford University Press and my two reviewers for their generous support of this book. Last but not least, special thanks to Roxi Copland for her continued willingness to put up with me on a daily basis.

AI	artificial intelligence
ALG-P	Algorithmic Pain Prediction
AUC	area under the curve
AUROC	area under the receiver operating curve
CCC	Lin's concordance correlation coefficient
CONSORT	Consolidated Standards for Reporting of Trials
CRT	Critical Race Theory
DCNN	deep convoluted neural network
DNN	deep neural network
DTC	direct-to-consumer
EHR	electronic health records
EIS	environmental impact statement
ERB	ethics review board
FN	false negative
FNAC	fine needle aspiration cytology
FONSI	finding of no significant impact
FP	false positive
ICC	intra-class correlation coefficient
IRB	Institutional Review Board
JITAI	just-in-time adaptive interventions
KLG	Kellgren–Lawrence Grade
KNN	k-nearest neighbor algorithm
MCI	mild cognitive impairment

MeSH	medical subject headings
MI-CLAIM	minimum information about clinical artificial intelligence modeling
ML	machine learning
MMSE	Mini Mental State Examination
NEPA	National Environmental Policy Act
NPRS	Numeric Pain Rating Scale
PPGR	postprandial (post-meal) glycemic responses
R-CNN	regional convoluted neural network
ROC	receiver operating characteristic
RS	rough set theory
RSNA	Radiology Society of North America
SDoH	social determinants of health
SPIRIT	standard reporting for interventional trials
STS	Science and Technology Studies
SVM	support vector machine
TN	true negative
TNR	true negative rate
TP	true positive
TPLC	total product life cycle
TPR	true positive rate
VAS	Visual Analog Scale
WBCD	Wisconsin Breast Cancer Dataset
WMD	weapon of math destruction
XAI	eXplainable AI

Introduction

Promise and Peril in Health AI

> *[W]e are living in the Fourth Industrial Age, a revolution so pro-*
> *found that it may not be enough to compare it to the invention of*
> *steam power, the railroads, electricity, mass production, or even*
> *the computer age in the magnitude of change it will bring. . . . This*
> *revolution will overtake every human endeavor, medicine not least*
> *among them.*
>
> —ABRAHAM VERGHESE, Foreword to *Deep Medicine*

Reginald went to his primary care provider with blurred vision, dizziness, palpitations, and a stinging sensation in his lower spine. His doctor was not particularly surprised by this list of symptoms. She was well acquainted with Reginald's long history of hypochondria and generalized anxiety disorder. As she'd anticipated, there were no obvious signs of illness or injury upon examination. At worst, Reginald had a mild case of the flu, and so she sent him away with some antibiotics bordering on placebo. It was not much longer before Reginald's symptoms started to progress. His anxiety and general sense of unease were followed by more obvious symptoms including sudden-onset scleroderma and hyperpigmentation (thickening and darkening of the skin). The subsequent legions and pustules on the chest and face were enough to get Reginald some more serious medical attention. In the end, it would take cutting-edge artificial intelligence (AI)

The Doctor and the Algorithm. S. Scott Graham, Oxford University Press. © Oxford University Press 2022.
DOI: 10.1093/oso/9780197644461.003.0001

and precision genomics to identify the cause of Reginald's illness and to develop an appropriate treatment plan. Sophisticated sorting algorithms were able to sift through millions of DNA base pairs to identify a previously unknown genetic mutation that was responsible for what would turn out to be an emerging autoimmune condition. Although there had been no preexisting treatment options available, another AI system was able to leverage the latest advances in precision genomics to determine a successful therapeutic approach. Where a tired, overworked, and perhaps inattentive physician missed the correct diagnosis, AI was able to save the day.

Stories like this one are stock-in-trade for medical futurists and AI evangelists. You can read countless tales of overworked or biased human and failed healthcare systems that are outperformed by the latest advances in machine learning, deep neural networks, and precision medicine. In fact, Reginald's tale is almost identical to a motivating narrative in Eric Topol's *Deep Medicine*.[1] Topol tells the story of an apparently healthy newborn who suddenly developed unexplained seizures. After all the normal tests failed to lead to a diagnosis . . .

> a blood sample was sent to Rady's Genomic Institute for a rapid whole-genome sequencing. The sequence encompassed 125 gigabytes of data, including nearly 5 million locations where the child's genome differed from the most common one. It took twenty seconds for a form of AI called natural-language processing to ingest the boy's electronic medical record and determine eighty-eight phenotype features (almost twenty times more than the doctors had summarized in their problem list). Machine-learning algorithms quickly sifted the approximately 4 million genetic variants to find the roughly 700,000 rare ones. Of those, 962 are known to cause disease. Combining that information with the boy's phenotypic data, the system identified one, in a gene called ADLH7A, as the most likely culprit.[2]

The major difference between Topol's vignette and the one at the outset of this book is that Reginald's story is fiction. It is the plot of a 1994

Star Trek: The Next Generation episode, and poor Reginald is actually de-evolving into some sort of ancestral spider species. The AIs who save him are, of course, the ship's computer and an android, Lieutenant Commander Data.

As a scholar of rhetoric, I am trained to see patterns in language and argument. But you don't need a Ph.D. in rhetoric to appreciate the strong parallels between the promotional narratives of health AI and the stories of science fiction. These similarities are not just an interesting coincidence. In fact, they may be a real cause for concern. If the stories we use to justify health AI are indistinguishable from science fiction, then it's a critical matter for us to assess whether (a) today's technology has really eclipsed 1994's imagination of the 24th century, *or* whether (b) we are being sold a promise that AI cannot deliver. If it is the former, then this truly is an exciting time for medicine, and we can be enthusiastic about an impending revolution in care. If it is the latter, then we need to be on guard against the many potential negative consequences of embracing a tech fix that will not and cannot pay promised dividends. In short, this is a question of how we separate the hype from the reality. The question is simple. The answer, not so much.

Nevertheless, the goal of *The Doctor and the Algorithm* is to tackle this question head-on to try to provide something like answers. When it comes to the promise of health AI, we are facing a complex and rapidly unfolding situation. AI enthusiasts and critics alike talk about AI summers and AI winters. That is, over the course of the last 80 years, there have been intervening periods of AI enthusiasm and AI contempt/neglect. Relatively recent advances in machine learning combined with ever-increasing computational speeds in smaller, less expensive packages have led to a particularly hot AI summer of late. Well-known technologies like search engine algorithms, news aggregators, social media feeds, and self-driving cars are all part of the current AI summer. In academia and investigative journalism, the many dangers associated with these new technologies have catalyzed broad engagement with critical algorithm studies. Indeed, the work of Safiya Noble, Meredith Broussard, Cathy O'Neil, Ruha Benjamin, Thomas Mullaney, Benjamin Peters, Mar Hicks, Kavita Philip, and many

others now offers a much-needed counterweight to the unbridled AI enthusiasm of Silicon Valley. The efforts of these scholars and journalists
may even presage a new AI winter. But that winter is not here yet, and
many technology sectors remain quite enthusiastic about embracing AI.
In recent years, we have seen a similar proliferation of health AI focused
on diagnosis, prognosis, healthcare systems management, drug discovery,
disease modeling, and so on. On the one hand, the promises of deep medicine are scintillating, and there is great potential for improved health
outcomes. On the other hand, the many cautionary tales of AI, more
broadly, suggest that we should be wary.

For the most part, there are three kinds of books about AI: (1) technical literature, including scientific reports and how-to guides, (2) techno-
futurist evangelism that champions the never-ending promise of AI, and
(3) horror tours—unrelenting explorations of the damage done by AI.[3]
The Doctor and the Algorithm will not be any of these kinds of books.
It's definitely not a technical manual. It also won't be techno-futurism.
That book already exists several times over. We don't need another one,
and I'm not that optimistic about the promise of health AI. There is certainly a version of this book that could be more traditional critical algorithm studies. I'm honestly tempted to embrace one of Thomas Mullaney's
playful caricatures of critical algorithm scholars as "gadflies . . . always
dwelling upon the negative" or "millenarian street preachers waving signs
that read 'The End is Nigh.'"[4] These are comfortable roles for me as a critical humanities scholar, and it would not be too difficult to curate a spate
of horror stories featuring health AI gone wrong. However, *The Doctor
and the Algorithm* is not going to be that book either. To put my cards on
the table, I'm "AI—cautiously optimistic." I believe that AI has a lot to offer
when used carefully, appropriately, and ethically. There are some undoubt-
edly promising advances in health AI. What's more, I even use AI in my
own scholarship and will use AI to explore health AI hype in *The Doctor
and the Algorithm*. All that said, I am mindful of the many limitations and
dangers that AI presents. I tend to agree with Mullaney that the (mis)use
of AI is an emergency requiring immediate intervention.[5] And so, *The
Doctor and the Algorithm* aims to live up to its subtitle—*Promise, Peril,*

and the Future of Health AI. My goal is to carefully explore the promise and the peril—both of which are often manifest in exactly the same AI systems.

THE PROMISE

The promises offered on behalf of health AI do not get much clearer than the opening epigraph to this book. A "Fourth Industrial Age" that surpasses "steam power, the railroads, electricity, mass production, or even the computer age" is an extraordinarily high bar to clear. It is a wonder Verghese didn't include fire or the wheel on his list of lesser accomplishments. While I'm wearing my gadfly hat here, it's important to note how serious Verghese and Topol are. They are not isolated prognosticators but, rather, authoritative voices from academic medicine. Abraham Verghese is a professor of medicine at Stanford University. And Eric Topol worked at several university medical schools before founding Scripps Research, a nonprofit medical research institute. Perhaps most notably, he has received over $200 million in grant funding from the National Institutes of Health (NIH) to advance deep medicine in the United States. Given his status as a leading clinical researcher, we would be remiss if we did not take Topol seriously when he claims, "AI in medicine isn't just a futuristic premise. The power of AI is already being harnessed to help save lives."[6] So, if Star Trek's 1994 vision of health AI is practically here already, just what can deep medicine do?

A good place to start in answering this question is a recently published edited collection, *Artificial Intelligence in Medicine: Technical Basis and Clinical Applications*.[7] As the title suggests, this is that first kind of health AI book—technical literature. The volume includes 25 chapters and essays by many leading academic and industry health technologists. The collected contributions serve a range of purposes from outlining future research agendas to reporting on efforts to develop specific new AI systems. Despite the more circumspect tone of an academic volume, the identified potentials of AI remain expansive. As the introduction illustrates,

Benefits of AI in medicine extend across multiple axes: (1) As already mentioned, AI can be applied across the spectrum of basic to translational research and clinical practice. (2) Within clinical practice AI applications extend across settings and health-care access points—from everyday home and work environments to the family practitioner's office, the emergency room, the hospital ward, operating room, intensive care unit. (3) AI benefits extend across the lifespan from preconception and pregnancy planning to end-of-life care.[8]

If we can accept these promises at face value, AI has the potential to radically improve gamete-to-grave medicine, transforming essentially all aspects of care and health system delivery. As the Introduction authors make their case, they outline several more specific benefits that we can reasonably expect AI to bring to medicine soon. These include improvements in diagnostic accuracy, increases in healthcare system efficiency, broadening access to care, and turbocharging preventative medicine through predictive analytics.

Importantly, the promise of health AI is not limited to discrete clinical encounters. AI technologies are optimized for predictive analytics and thus have significant potential beyond individual patients. One non-clinical area receiving a lot of attention is public health. Over the course of the COVID-19 pandemic, we have seen the results of many AI systems in forecasting of disease spread, fatality rates, and potential mutations. Broadly, AI-driven public health surveillance aims to identify "early, accurate, and reliable signals of health anomalies and disease outbreaks from a heterogeneous collection of data sources . . . "[9] Another nonclinical area generating significant excitement involves using AI for drug discovery. Researchers are actively developing AI systems that dredge and aggregate complex chemical data and subsequently recommend existing or novel compounds that might serve as suitable drugs. University of Cambridge systems biologist Steve Oliver goes so far as to suggest that "Robot scientists using AI can test more compounds, and do so with improved accuracy and reproducibility, and exhaustive, searchable record-keeping."[10] The compound BPM31510 is one such AI-identified option for treating a variety of cancers.[11] The drug is currently undergoing clinical trials for use in pancreatic cancer, glioblastoma, and squamous cell carcinoma. The hope is that BPM31510 will prove safe and effective for patients who have responded poorly or had serious adverse reactions to other chemotherapy agents in the past.[12]

But the question of what we can accept at face value remains a vexing one. Even Topol's *Deep Medicine* includes a list of "outlandish expectations for AI." He notes that many suggest AI will:

> Outperform doctors at all tasks; diagnose the undiagnosable; treat the untreatable; see the unseeable on scans, slides; predict the unpredictable; classify the unclassifiable; eliminate workflow inefficiencies; eliminate hospital admissions and readmissions; eliminate the surfeit of unnecessary jobs; 100% medication adherence; zero patient harm; cure cancer.[13]

Certainly, there will never be "zero patient harm" or "100% medication adherence," yet the rhetoric of medical futurism hints at these kinds of things as real possible futures. Despite dubbing each of these promises "outlandish," Topol eventually vouches for many of them in the pages of *Deep Medicine*. For example, later chapters in *Deep Medicine* provide a litany of examples where AI outperforms humans and occasionally even exhibits "superhuman performance."[14] In the end, Topol offers a bold, speculative vision for deep medicine, a vision he justifies based on the potential for rapid accurate diagnoses, precision customized treatment plans, the elimination of economic inefficiencies (which, in large part, seems to mean nurses),[15] and a new foundation of empathy for the practice of medicine. That last part is especially tricky. Essentially, Topol argues that when AI frees physicians from the administrative burdens of electronic medical records, reading lab results, and performing analyses, then they will be better able to provide patients with the emotional labor so often lacking in contemporary medicine.

Fourth Industrial Age or not, there are real reasons to be excited about the potential of deep medicine. Even modest reductions in medical error rates, limited improvements in diagnostic accuracy, and slightly more rapid outbreak detection could result in significant improvements in health and even save lives. If it is remotely possible that AI might offer these benefits, then the technology seems worth exploring further. Of course, caution must be a guiding principle. Critical algorithm studies have taught us that there are many dangers alongside the potential. AI development is driven significantly by "self-confidence . . . self-assurance . . . [and] 'bias toward action.'"[16] In short, the AI community has been quick to believe its own hype, and the result has been the overly enthusiastic adoption of dangerous and damaging technologies. Carefully investigating the promise of health AI requires being assiduously attentive to the many perils. If improvements in care are not broadly distributed, then deep medicine will reinforce and exacerbate long-standing health inequities and injustices. Adopting new medical technologies is always a question of risk–benefit ratios. But a recurrent challenge is assuring that we are mindful of broader risks and negative externalities that extend beyond those commonly detected by carefully designed clinical trials. To keep these potential perils front and center, I now turn to an exploration of the many perils of AI both within and beyond healthcare.

THE PERIL

As mentioned above, much has been written in recent years documenting the dangers of AI, especially in non-medical contexts. For example, Ruha Benjamin's *Race after Technology*[17] and Safiya Noble's *Algorithms of Oppression*[18] offer particularly harrowing insights about the perils and pitfalls of AI. Benjamin and Noble detail the many pernicious ways that AI-driven search engines, facial recognition, social media, credit scoring, and predictive policing further inflict racism on already marginalized communities. In *Algorithms of Oppression* Noble offers a deep dive into how racism and misogyny are reified, reinforced, and manifested through search engine technologies. One of Noble's opening vignettes is particularly striking. As she writes, "While googling things on the Internet that might be interesting to my stepdaughter and nieces, I was overtaken by the results. My search on the keywords 'black girls' yielded HotBlackPussy.com as the first hit. Hit indeed."[19] Ultimately, Noble documents how evolving search engine algorithms prioritize a heteronormative white male gaze that overlaps substantively with the demographics of Google's developers and engineers. Pornography results have been routinely returned when search terms reference Black and brown people, but not for "white girls." The search engine's autocomplete predictive text has prompted users to ask why Black women are so angry, loud, mean, attractive, lazy, annoying, sassy, and insecure. While Google has done much to correct these issues, it is horrifying that these kinds of results were ever possible on a live release of their signature product.

Benjamin's *Race after Technology* explores a broader range of technologies under the purview of "the New Jim Code: the employment of new technologies that reflect and produce existing inequities but that are promoted and perceived as more objective or progressive than the discriminatory systems of a previous era."[20] Ultimately, Benjamin documents how algorithms in banking, criminal justice, pre-employment screening, social media, and so on aggregate and concretize racism. The implicit biases and structural racism of training data cannot help but produce algorithms that perpetuate and reinforce discrimination, all while being packaged in claims to objectivity and non-bias. As she notes,

The danger of New Jim Code impartiality is the neglect of ongoing inequity perpetuated by colorblind designs. In this context, algorithms may not be just a veneer that covers historical fault lines. They also seem to be streamlining discrimination—making it easier to sift, sort, and justify why tomorrow's workforce continues to be racially stratified. Algorithmic neutrality reproduces algorithmically sustained discrimination.[21]

As Benjamin notes, deferring judgment to cold, unthinking mathematical machines essentially creates what Eduardo Bonilla-Silva calls "racism without racists."[22] The math hides the bias and in so doing deflects responsibility.

One of the reasons AI is so prone to hype despite obvious failings is that the rhetoric of AI tends to treat *quantitization* as quantification. To quantify implies measurement, accuracy, precision. Quantification assumes that the values we assign are indexed to an objective reality or at least an agreed-upon standard. To quantitize, on the other hand, is merely to assign a number. A simple example will serve to make the point. The actor Matthew McConaughey teaches a film class where I work at the University of Texas at Austin. Every once in a blue moon, I see him around campus. I'm taller than Matthew McConaughey, but not by much. We can quantify this. He's 6'0", and on a good day, I'm 6'½". Even though I'm a bit taller, Matthew McConaughey is arguably more attractive than I am. Let's say he's a rugged 9.5 out of 10, and I'm . . . well . . . not. Here we've quantitized a subjective evaluation of attractiveness. It's not wrong, but it's not precise, accurate, or universal. If we were to call this quantification instead of quantitization, we would be implying a higher standard of accuracy than actually exists.

Now, obviously, the stakes of treating quantitization as quantification are a lot more serious than the extent to which Matthew McConaughey is more attractive than I am. Indeed, this is one of the primary issues driving Cathy O'Neil's analysis of "Weapons of Math Description" or WMDs.[23] O'Neil's WMD analytic is broader than just bad AI. She uses the concept to describe a wide variety of problematic quantitization regimes including subprime mortgage valuation, *US News & World Report* college rankings, and poorly designed teacher assessment metrics. As O'Neil describes WMDs,

[M]any of these models encoded human prejudice, misunderstanding, and bias into the software systems that increasingly managed our lives. Like gods, these mathematical models were opaque, their workings invisible to all but the highest priests in their domain: mathematicians and computer scientists. Their verdicts, even when wrong or harmful were beyond dispute or appeal. And they ended to punish the poor and the oppressed in our society, while making the rich richer.[24]

On the whole, *Weapons of Math Destruction* offers an insider's perspective of unethical quantitization regimes: credit scoring, digital redlining, predictive policing, social media manipulation, and so on. When combined with the insights of Benjamin and Noble, a very dismal picture of AI starts to emerge.

Now, this is a book about *health* AI, so you might be wondering why I'm spending so much time on search engines, social media, credit scoring, and predictive policing. The simple answer is because it's the same. AI in health and other tech sectors are identical at both digital and material levels. The convolutional neural networks, nearest-neighbor algorithms, and support vector machines of the New Jim Code are literally the same computational libraries as those used in precision diagnostics and automated clinical note taking. What's more: new advances in health AI are often developed and promulgated by the very same companies that have had so many issues in other sectors. Google's DeepMind is an industry leader in health AI, yet there's little reason to suspect that the health division operates so differently from the search engine division that it is immune to implicit biases. Topol's *Deep Medicine* celebrates the story of Eric Lefkosky, the Groupon founder who, despite having "no science background," was "perplexed at how little data permeated [cancer] care."[25] Lefkosky subsequently launched Tempus Labs, an exercise in venture capital and disruptive innovation, now another industry leader in health AI. Even when health AI development is not occurring in literally the same Silicon Valley spaces, much in the way of medical futurism it looks toward deeper integration with Big Tech. Disturbingly, *Deep Medicine* also enthusiastically describes efforts to integrate mental health analytics and automated psychotherapy with Weibo and Facebook.[26]

Finally, medicine itself (even without AI) is certainly not without biases. A 2016 survey of 121 medical trainees found that 58% believed that Black skin is thicker than white skin.[27] All in all, 73% respondents endorsed at least one false statement about biological differences by race. These implicit biases have real and deleterious effects on patient care. Physicians who endorsed false beliefs about biological differences were significantly more likely to under-assess pain in Black patients. These data add significant nuance to long documented issues where Black patients are less likely to receive appropriate pain care in terms of diagnostic X-rays and necessary opiate pharmacology compared with white patients.

Structural racism and implicit biases have also been shown to affect technological development in health and medicine (even before the advent of AI). Benjamin's *Race after Technology* tells the story of the spirometer, a device that measures lung capacity.[28] Presumptions of differential physiology are so embedded in healthcare that the spirometer has a button that changes the measurements for Black patients. The racism of the spirometer has real material effects not only on healthcare delivery, but significantly in the context of workers' compensation related to asbestos liability. Recalibration by race

made it more difficult for Black workers to qualify for workers' compensation. Black workers were required to demonstrate worse lung function and more severe clinical symptoms than White workers owing to this feature of the spirometer, whose developer, Dr. John Hutchinson, was employed by insurance companies in the mid-1800s to minimize payouts.[29]

While some might want to gloss over this as a case of medicine corrupted by the insurance industry, such a move risks ignoring the many ways the economics of medicine transform the practice of medicine.

More recently, COVID-19 has forced healthcare providers to confront a serious issue of bias in one of the most common medical technologies—pulse oximetry. A pulse oximeter, or "pulse ox" as it is commonly called, is a seemingly elegant diagnostic tool for measuring oxygen saturation in the bloodstream. A small plastic clip attaches to the patient's finger and projects a red light bright enough to be detectable all the way through the finger. Oxygen-saturated hemoglobin generally appears red, which means that it reflects red wavelengths of light. Deoxygenated blood appears darker and reflects infrared or near infrared light. A pulse ox detects how much red and infrared light makes it through the finger in order to infer oxygen saturation levels based on a double ratio of the two wavelengths. As you may have already guessed, pulse oximetry was developed primarily using white patients. As a result, the calculations that evaluate how much of what kind of light passes through a finger are not accurate for Black patients. The error is magnified at low oxygen saturation levels, and this led directly to higher mortality rates for Black patients during the COVID-19 pandemic. Pulse ox technology (developed on white skin) overestimates oxygen saturation for Black patients, and this overestimation results in delayed oxygen support (mask, ventilation, intubation). Any such delays are a serious problem for COVID patients, who can crash quickly without proper oxygen support.

WHAT IF THE HYPE IS RIGHT?

An important caveat in *Weapons of Math Destruction* is that not all quantitative or computational systems qualify as WMDs. O'Neal points to sabermetrics or moneyball as one example of quantification that is not a quantitization. Sabermetrics is baseball statistics. It is the careful use of player data (hits, home runs, walks, etc.) and predictive modeling to curate high-scoring low-cost teams. Historically, fielding a winning baseball team has been based on the art of scouting. Recruiters with long experience look for outstanding high school and college players. Then teams compete over signing them based on offering ever-increasing piles of money. Sabermetrics was originally developed as an academic exercise in a series of papers published between 1977 and 1988 by Bill James. The most famous successful use case for sabermetrics was the 2002 Oakland Athletics, a story that is the basis behind the Brad Pitt and Jonah Hill film *Moneyball* (as well as the book of the same name). Long story short, A's manager Billy Beane didn't have a big enough budget to compete effectively in player recruitment. So Beane leveraged sabermetrics to identify "discount" players who could produce many runs even though they didn't have the "it" factor that scouts were looking for. O'Neal suggests that sabermetric models aren't WMDs because they are transparent, don't reply on surrogate measures, and are constantly updated based on new data. As she describes it,

> Baseball also has statistical rigor. Its gurus have an immense data set at hand, almost all of it directly related to the performance of players in the game. Moreover, their data is highly relevant to the outcomes they are trying to predict. . . . Most crucially, that data is constantly pouring in, with new statistics from an average of twelve or thirteen games arriving daily from April to October. Statistics can compare the results of these games to the predictions of their models and they can see where they were wrong. . . . That's how trustworthy models operate. They maintain a constant back-and-forth with whatever in the world they're trying to understand or predict. Conditions change, and so must the model.[30]

As mentioned above, there's reason to think that at least *some* health AI might be like sabermetrics. That is, biomedical publishing, federal regulation, and patient health outcomes have the potential to provide the right mix of transparency and ongoing model refinement such that we can trust the claims of health AI.

I have never seen Gmail's spam filter confusion matrix, but I've seen many in medical journals. A confusion matrix is a data table used to assess the performance of an AI system. To determine how often an AI gets it "right," developers apply the AI to a data set where the answers are already known. So, if the system is designed to flag spam, the engineers feed a bunch of examples of known spam and known legitimate email to the system. In comparing the AI guesses (spam vs. not spam) to what is already known about each email, you can create a confusion matrix that documents the number of true positives (AI says spam, and it is spam), true negatives (AI says not spam, and it's not spam), false positives (AI says spam, but it's not spam), and false negatives (AI says not spam, but it is). Gmail is a black box. I have no idea how well it performs, even though I think it does a pretty good job (with spam detection). In contrast, I can quickly extract the confusion matrix data from many health AI studies. Even when these data are not reported in the published literature, they are generally required to be reported to the FDA before a new diagnostic system can be approved for broad usage.[31]

As O'Neil points out, when a bank gets it wrong, they often have no idea. If an automated credit scoring decision denies credit based on racist or specious data, the lender will never know. Maybe the customer finds credit with another institution that uses better practices. More likely, the customer suffers an injustice without possibility of repair. In either case, the bank has no way to improve their model based on this failure. When a doctor gets it wrong, people get hurt, sick, and/or die. There is plenty of potential injustice in this situation to be sure, but there is also a feedback loop that can lead to model improvement. Hospital systems regularly conduct mortality and morbidity reviews—retrospective assessments of deaths and injuries to improve future practice. The FDA maintains an Adverse Events Reporting System (FAERS) where healthcare providers can (and in some cases are required to) provide details on patient side effects, serious illness or injury, and even deaths associated with regulated products. FAERS is an important part of "post-marketing surveillance," the FDA's efforts to continually monitor approved drugs and devices. These are just a few quick examples of the ways in which it is possible for health AI systems to escape the pitfalls of WMDs. Certainly, not all medical AI systems successfully do so. Nevertheless, it seems possible that when (1) developed systems are engineered using gold standard measures, (2) results are communicated openly and transparently, and (3) systems are refined through diligent post-marketing surveillance, they just might live up to the promises of health AI.

HYPE, PROMISE, AND PERIL

According to the folks at Merriam-Webster, to hype is "to promote or publicize extravagantly." Dictionaries provide a sense of everyday usage of a word, but they are not exhaustive of meaning. The typical default conception of hype relies on "extravagance." Following this definition, when we see grandiose claims like "The Fourth Industrial Age," we quite reasonably assume hype. But promotional language and extravagance do not really exhaust the full meaning of "hype." In one study of scientific press releases and corresponding news articles, the authors gloss hype as "exaggerate[ing] the importance of a scientific finding."[32] That *exaggeration* part is key. Hype is not just promotional language. It is promotional language that promises more than can be delivered. In this context, it becomes possible to imagine an extravagant promotional language that does not equal hype. This is another way of suggesting we ask, "What if the 'hype' is right?" Even careful metanalyses of diagnostic AI show that new technologies are, indeed, equaling and even outperforming doctors in some cases. If AI really is more accurate, is it fair to call it hype? I'm still not ready to double-down on the idea that deep medicine will be more transformative than electricity, but it's absolutely worth taking seriously the idea that health AI may well not be all hype.

As mentioned above, addressing this question is the central purpose of *The Doctor and the Algorithm*. In so doing, this book will proceed by exploring the sociotechnical systems that make and promulgate AI, the methodological and philosophical foundations for AI's promissory claims, the nature and extent of hype in deep medicine, the ways AI seeks to transform medicine itself, and possible regulatory frameworks for a just approach to deep medicine. These initiatives are spread across seven chapters, each focusing on key concepts and real-world examples from health AI. Here, I will close with a preview of these chapters and a few details about the broader interconnecting themes of *The Doctor and the Algorithm*.

Deep Medicine's Sociotechnical Systems

AI development in deep medicine is embedded in multifaceted sociotechnical systems that involve not only cutting-edge advances in computer science and medicine, but also scientific standards, regulatory structures, and economic systems. Algorithms and neural networks find patterns in numeric vectors, and AI accuracy is measured following one of several conflicting approaches established by federal regulation and/or relevant disciplines. Despite the highly technical nature of these practices, they are also inherently social. Thus, AI development is a complex choreography of humans and technology, and to understand deep medicine is to understand how sociotechnical systems cohere, conflict, and continue. Untangling these systems is the primary aim of Chapter 1, "How to Make an AI." The chapter offers an orientation to the technical details of AI development and explores how the many systems that compose AI are assembled into a single package or product. Along the way, Chapter 1 also reflects on how bias can enter the sociotechnical systems of deep medicine in different ways at different moments in the AI development process. Building on Chapter 1's exploration of these different risk vectors, Chapter 2, "Digital Oracles," shifts attention to medical futurism and efforts to fundamentally transform and reshape medicine's current sociotechnical systems through advances in AI. Emerging technologies are offered up with the aim of shifting the fundamental logics of medicine, health, and care. As I argue in Chapter 2, accepting these proposed shifts requires investing significant (and often misplaced) trust in new digital systems. Thus, in closing this chapter, I reflect on the extent to which misplaced trust fuels what Broussard calls "technochauvinism"[33] in some areas of deep medicine.

Hype in Deep Medicine

Chapter 3, "How to Make It as an AI," describes the many continuities between AI development and dissemination, promulgation, and promotion. Success in AI is about building systems that are responsive to the full range of sociotechnical system pressures. Scientific standards, clinical commitments, regulatory structures, and economic incentives collide to create a fraught landscape for just AI development and popularization. In so doing, Chapter 3 explores in more detail how accuracy claims become the foundation of promotional claims and trust in AI (misplaced or otherwise). That is, successful AI systems in deep medicine are said to be accurate based on the extent to which predictions made match "ground truth." Despite the term, ground truth is seldom just found conveniently lying around. So, Chapter 4, "The Search for Ground Truth," investigates the ways that ground truth must be dredged up, engineered, or forged by the architects of AI systems. In these cases, "accuracy" becomes a sophisticated deferral where agreement between two systems is taken for truth. This is the ideal environment for hype—both accidental and intentional. Along the way, Chapter 4 offers an exercise inspired by public interest informatics and data feminism.[34] Specifically, I create and explore a simulation that models the search for ground truth and exposes serious limitations in the most common research designs. Next, Chapter 5, "HypeDx," investigates the complex interrelationships of promotional claims about health AI in scientific, media, and public relations venues. More specifically, Chapter 5 details the failures of the "two-stage" model of scientific dissertation that imagines an initial stage of dispassionate scientific inquiry followed by a subsequent stage of marketing and promotion. In exploring hype in deep medicine, I have developed my own AI systems that identify and classify both promotional and hedged language in biomedical research. HypeDX and HedgeDX, as I call them, leverage advances in machine learning and natural language processing so as to classify promotional and hedging language about health AI with near-human precision (Oops—did I just hype myself?). These systems allow me to explore the prevalence of promotional language in published research on health AI and to identify research reports at the greatest risk of exaggeration.

Better Health AI

As we become increasingly aware of the dangers of AI, we are seeing a proliferation of new initiatives designed to promote better AI. Chapter 6, "Ethics, Justice, and Health AI," explores the differences between (1) Ethical

AI's focus on regulation and audits, and (2) Just AI's focus on precaution or explicitly emancipatory intervention. With reference to case studies in AI-based pain measurement, the chapter addresses the fraught ethical and clinical landscapes created by efforts to use technology to address racism and ableism in medicine. Additionally, inventors and entrepreneurs in deep medicine are pursuing new uses of AI at a pace with which regulatory agencies struggle to keep up. Accordingly, in January 2021, the FDA released a proposed regulatory framework and discussion paper designed to catalyze improvements in health AI regulation. Chapter 7, "Regulating Health AI," explores this proposal in the context of best-practice recommendations from advocates for just and ethical AI. Finally, the pursuit of ethical and just AI cannot merely be an exercise in retrospective evaluation. It is critical that we develop social and regulatory frameworks that support and encourage ethical development and just applications. This will require the coordinated efforts of academics, researchers, journals, activists, journalists, legislators, and regulators. Subsequently, *The Doctor and the Algorithm* will close with a chapter that aims to move in this direction: "Conclusion: Just Futures for Deep Medicine." In this chapter, I explore emerging initiatives that might support a future for deep medicine that better lives up to the current promises.

How to Make an AI

If you want to house-train your dog, you have to let her pee in your house. It is an unfortunate paradox, but true all the same. If you keep a dog crated up or outside all the time, she will never have the chance to pee inside and receive that gentle correction from which learning stems. Housetraining, like most leaning processes, relies on a mix of praise and correction until the lesson sticks. When you have a new dog, you must be ever vigilant. Whether you're making dinner, watching TV, or working from home, you always need to have one eye on your new furry friend. The second she starts to assume the position, you spring into action, offer a firm "No!," and escort her quickly outside. With luck, she will finish doing her business outside, and you can shift from correction to praise: "You're such a good dog! Such a good dog. Here's a cookie!"

We have a froston (half French bulldog, half Boston terrier) named Odin. Odin is smart, but stubborn. This was a real issue during housetraining. Because she's smart, she never peed in the same place a second time after being told not to. But because she's smart and also stubborn, she had to systematically rule out every possible pee place in the house. Seriously— she would pee in the hallway. You'd yell, "No!," and do the whole outside/positive reinforcement thing. Then the next day, she would pee five feet down the hall. The next day five feet further, and so on. A process of elimination for her processes of elimination, if you will. As any dog companion will tell you, 100% perfection takes time. About seven years later, we got another dog named Haggis. Now, let's say I were to make a map

The Doctor and the Algorithm. S. Scott Graham, Oxford University Press. © Oxford University Press 2022.
DOI: 10.1093/oso/9780197644461.003.0002

of all the places Odin peed and was corrected and all the places Odin peed and was rewarded. Let's also say instead of housetraining Haggis the old-fashioned way, I could show the map to her, and she'd instantly be housetrained about as well as Odin was. Wouldn't that be amazing? As you may have already surmised, that's AI. Housetraining is about finding a line. It is teaching your dog to recognize the division between inside and outside. In the middle of the housetraining process, it is not always clear where that line is. Odin knew the first five feet of the hallway were off limits, so she tried the next five feet, and the next five feet until she found the line. There are many different kinds of AI out there. However, quite a few literally find a line. Designing an AI is about creating something like a map. That map is sent to an algorithm (a specially designed set of computer instructions) that finds the line in the map. See Figure 1.1.

Most AI right now is the result of machine learning (ML), and ML-based binary classification is a great place to start for our tour of health AI. My extended exercise in housetraining is a typical example of binary classification. I detail the processes involved in teaching a dog to recognize two different types of spaces (good pee places and bad pee places). Usually

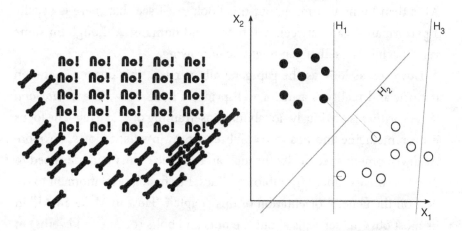

Figure 1.1. Map of housetraining successes and failures (left) and a toy model support vector machine (SVM) binary classifier (right) where H2 is the most efficient dividing line between data classes.

SOURCE: Cyc, Graphic showing 3 Hyperplanes in 2D, 2008, https://commons.wikimedia.org/wiki/File:Svm_separating_hyperplanes.png.

when people think of AI, they think something like "machines that do smart things." This is both true and not true. Science fiction portrayals of AI often feature computers that can do many things very well. Star Trek's Lieutenant Commander Data, mentioned in the Introduction, does basically everything well. He's better than humans at science, engineering, combat arts, chess, playing the violin, and even—apparently—sex.[1] In contrast, contemporary (and real) AI usually involves using a machine-learning algorithm to teach a computer to do one specific thing (don't pee in the house!). As Efstathios Gennatas and Jonathan Chen of Stanford University Medical School note in their introduction to *Artificial Intelligence in Medicine*, "Currently popular forms of AI/ML algorithms largely operate on a single circumscribed task at a time."[2] A more accurate definition for most AI is probably something like "a machine that does one smart thing, but only kind of smartly." And like the dog training example, machine-learning-based AI is pretty good, but almost never as good as a human. I'm pretty happy with how well trained Odin and Haggis are, but they've both had more post-housetraining accidents than I have. Obviously, Odin and Haggis are dogs, and AIs are usually built with fancy computers. Nevertheless, despite all the rhetoric about how much better AI is than humans, throughout this book, we'll see that there is usually a performance gap between computers and humans. Although, in some very specific cases, that gap might be narrowing.

However, as long as the gap generally persists, this distance between rhetoric and reality is a major wellspring of hype. Now, *The Doctor and the Algorithm* is obviously not about housetraining or Star Trek. The focus is deep medicine and health AI. Subsequently, in what follows, I explore AI development specifically through an example of a system designed to diagnose breast cancer from biopsy slides. But first, a brief moment to reflect on the general orientation of this chapter. "How to Make an AI," in its most obvious sense, is about the nuts and bolts (or ones and zeros) of systems development. So, in what follows, I will spend a fair amount of time outlining the details of data curation, feature engineering, model selection, tuning parameters, and accuracy assessments. Each of these technical activities is central to making an AI.

BLACKBOXING IN SOCIOTECHNICAL SYSTEMS

Technical details are often where people start to explain AI. Indeed, "opening up the black box" is a common technique in science and technology studies (STS). The idea is to better understand the occluded machinations of technology and/or power. As Benjamin describes her project in *Race after Technology*,

> [T]his book employs a conceptual toolkit that synthesizes scholarship from STS and critical race studies. Surprisingly, these two fields of study are not often put into direct conversation. STS scholarship opens wide the "Black box" that typically conceals the inner workings of socio-technical systems, and critical race studies interrogates the inner workings of sociolegal systems.[3]

"Opening the black box," as a metaphorical and methodological move, is extraordinarily common. At the time of this writing "opening the black box" (in quotation marks) returns 33,600 results on Google Scholar. Ultimately, the black box metaphor is based on the idea that technological details are elided and sometimes even hidden behind a literal box, the opening of which voids warranties (or worse). Now, you may have noted that the section title here is not "opening the black box of health AI." It is the rather more awkward "Blackboxing in Sociotechnical Systems." The metaphor of *opening* the black box relies on the assumption of a ready-made and closed box that needs opening. This can be a perfectly appropriate methodological approach depending on when one engages with technical systems of interest. This approach fits well with Bruno Latour's early formulation of the black box in *Science in Action*. As he describes it, "The word black box is used by cyberneticians whenever a piece of machinery or a set of commands is too complex. In its place they draw a little box about which they need to know nothing but its input and output."[4] Here Latour describes the root of the metaphor, an actual practice of *drawing* a black box. As this metaphor is extended methodologically, he eventually lands on the following more formal definition: "When many elements are made to act as one, this is what I will now call a black box."[5]

The black box (an occluded system of many elements made to act as one) is exactly what Ruha Benjamin, Safiya Noble, Catherine O'Neil, Meredith Broussard, and Halcyon Lawrence[6] encounter when they interrogate search engine algorithms, credit scoring, predictive policing, or voice-activated digital assistants. These systems present as singular discrete entities, are occluded by intellectual property concerns, and are offered ready-made to the world. When I shift away from the notion of *the* black box, it is not to criticize the work of Benjamin, Noble, O'Neil, Broussard, Lawrence, or countless others who open black boxes. Rather, it is to recognize that we can engage much of health AI earlier in the development process. We can be there at the moment that the systems engineer draws that little box on the technical diagram. Let's think about that moment for a second. The systems engineer *draws* a box. This is an act, an action, a human doing. *Blackboxing* is a verb. In *Pandora's Hope*, Latour also gerundifies the black box: "blackboxing, a process that makes the joint production of actors and artifacts entirely opaque."[7] However, as I have noticed previously, blackboxing is not just a matter of occlusion. Rather, it is a central part of "the authorization and legitimization of a new technology."[8] What's more, blackboxing is a team sport; it is an active process of occlusion and re-occlusion. As Latour noted in 1987, "if there is no one to take [a black box] up, it stops and falls apart however many people may have taken it up however long before."[9]

Blackboxing (as occlusion, authorization, and re-authorization) is an ongoing process that serves to make AI. This process is deployed in complex sociotechnical systems that integrate the activities of many humans and nonhumans. As such, it is critically important to understand how blackboxing occurs and how, once made, black boxes persist in sociotechnical systems. Opening up black boxes is a great way to understand the effects of technical systems on the world. It is a tremendously useful approach to exploring the hidden machinations of power that are intentionally occluded by technological and corporate systems. Exploring blackbox*ing* in action, on the other hand, gets us out in front of some of these effects. It gives us an opportunity to think through how new technologies are deployed and disseminated before they are fully blackboxed. It also helps us see the gap between the hype and the underlying reality.

The processes of blackboxing, however, are not enough on their own to help us understand what it means to make an AI. Black boxes, once made, circulate in sociotechnical systems, and that circulation is also an essential part of how AI does what it does. At the outset of this subsection, I include a passage from Benjamin where she points to how her work takes place at the intersection of STS and critical race theory (CRT). CRT provides unparalleled critical purchase on the sociolegal systems in which black boxes circulate. In this chapter, I am inspired in part by CRT, but CRT is not the only framework that drives my inquiry. I also draw on feminist STS broadly and Catherine D'Ignazio and Lauren Klein's invocation of it in *Data Feminism*. Building on the long tradition of feminist STS, D'Ignazio and Klein articulate a vision for critical engagement with technology centered around "a way of thinking about data, both their uses and their limits, that is informed by direct experience, by commitment to action, and by intersectional feminist thought."[10] As they further note, data feminism involves more than traditional humanities inquiry. The practice is also driven by "mobilizing data science to push back against existing and unequal power structures and to work toward more just and equitable futures."[11] Much of my data mobilization efforts are described in future chapters. However, the general precepts of CRT, feminist STS, and data feminism ultimately guide my attempt to make sense of the sociotechnical networks in which AI is made. In what follows, I begin this inquiry through analyses designed to get at the very nature of blackboxing processes and the mechanisms by which black boxes circulate in sociotechnical systems.

As the wealth of research in critical algorithm studies shows us, AI is a complex amalgamation of sociotechnical systems. AIs are assemblages of concretized human judgments, implicit biases, algorithms, tuning parameters, supercomputers, and political/economic investments. Benjamin, Noble, O'Neal, Broussard, D'Ignazio and Klein, and others have shown us many ways these systems, partially by virtue of their occlusion, are granted so much power in the world. Critical algorithm studies typically begin work at a point of breakdown. That is, when the inequitable and/or racist effects of a technology become clear, it is time to unpack the black box. As mentioned above, my goal here is to explore the processes of blackboxing itself. Rather than unpack, my goal is to explore the packing. Thus, in what follows, I explore blackboxing in breast cancer detection. In many parts of this book, I have selected case studies because the technologies represented are mundane. That is, the technologies developed in these studies are not revolutionary advances in medicine. They will not remake medicine anew. Importantly, "mundane" does not mean "harm free." Like essentially all subsystems within inequitable structures, the cases studied here participate in and perpetuate inequity. In her analysis of AI in criminal justice, Benjamin notes that "computer systems are a part of the larger matrix of systemic racism. Just as legal codes are granted an allure of objectivity . . . there is an enormous system around computer codes, which hides the human biases involved in technical design."[12] Legal codes are not substantively different from diagnostic codes in this case, and in the same way health AI runs serious risks of reinscribing and reifying health inequity under the banner of objectivity and accuracy. I start with these more mundane case studies for a reason. The processes of blackboxing are largely the same whether the technology is mundane, world changing, or community destroying. That's part of the insidiousness, after all. AI often replicates inequity, but it can also supercharge it. Blackboxing is part of what allows that to happen.

BLACKBOXING ENGINES

Over the course of this book's Introduction and first chapter, you may have noticed a subtle shift in terminology. Whereas I started writing about "health AI," I'm now just as likely to use Topol's term "deep medicine." This shift is intentional. As a term, "health AI" signals primarily the technological aspects of AI-driven medicine's sociotechnical systems. That is, "health AI" focuses our attention on the machines. This is precisely the primary function of blackboxing. It concretizes sociotechnical systems and presents them as ready-made objects. "Deep medicine," in contrast, draws our attention to how the technical is embedded in the sociological, economic, and ethical systems of health and medicine. While I'm not sure how much I agree with Topol's optimistic portrayal of where deep medicine will go, the term's attention to AI as embedded in clinical, economic, and regulatory structures is quite useful as a way of attending to the dynamic interactions among the social and the technical. Within this framework, my exploration of blackboxing engines requires some concerted engagement with the technical, but my goal is also to elucidate how the technical is embedded in the social. In so doing, I will point toward some of the common vectors by which bias can be and often is propagated through the sociotechnical systems of deep medicine.

Currently, one of the most promising areas of deep medicine is diagnostic AI. All that potential hype about AI being as good or better than doctors is about whether the machine can determine (as well or better than doctors) whether we have a given disease. That's a yes/no question, or binary classification, in many cases. While the opening vignette about housetraining my dogs provides a useful introductory metaphor for binary classification in AI, it doesn't quite cover all the critical concepts necessary to understand the blackboxing engines of AI development. So, before I can dive into the details of diagnostic AI, I must first describe a few of the more foundational features of AI development. My goal here is to provide the bare-bones essentials necessary to understand blackboxing engines. AI is, of course, many things, and so my gloss will not cover every possible implementation or technological architecture. Most notably, the focus in this chapter is on what is known as *supervised* machine learning. Here, supervision means that the training data for the AI system have been previously labeled by humans. Like the housetraining example, I provided the classifications (good pee place, bad bee place). In diagnostic medicine, the labels for each case might be cancer or not cancer, benign or malignant. Regardless of the particulars of the class, supervised machine learning is essentially about replicating a human classification process at scale. It is about teaching a machine to make the same kinds of decisions that humans make, usually using the same data.

Ultimately, supervised machine learning typically involves four primary activities: (1) data curation, (2) feature engineering, (3) model training, and (4) benchmarking. As mentioned previously, each of these steps in the AI development cycle provides different possible avenues for bias by dint of the sociotechnical system's activities in each stage of the process. Importantly, while each of the four stages provides a possible vector for bias, those vectors are not always activated. An individual AI system might be multiply compromised by bias at each stage of development, or it might be essentially ethical. In most cases, however, there are elements of potential bias at one or two stages and no cause for concern at others. This is the fraught nature of deep medicine. Almost no system is all good or all bad. It's a complex trade-off of risks and rewards. The trick for ethical health AI, of course, is to ensure that most of the risks are distributed and that rewards largely accrue to the patient. To get better traction on the sociotechnical systems of data curation, feature engineering, modeling, and benchmarking, in what follows, I explore a specific example in diagnostic AI. After a short discussion of the clinical area, I describe the social-technical systems, the risks of bias, and the details of the specific case for each of the major stages of AI development.

A CASE IN CANCER DIAGNOSTICS

Cancers are the second leading cause of death in the United States.[13] While "cancer" is usually discussed in the singular, I have made it plural here to help highlight the complexity of the situation for diagnostic AI. Cancers, in the aggregate, are the second most common cause of death nationally, but these deaths result from a wide range of malignancies. Ultimately, cancers are genetic mutations that cause certain cells to continue to divide rapidly and ad infinitum. The expanding clumps of cells become tumors, and if left unchecked they can metastasize or spread around the body. Colloquially, we usually classify cancer by location (skin, lung, breast), but oncologists are more likely to talk about tissue and cell types. The more technical taxonomy for cancer (sarcoma, myeloma, fibroadenoma, etc.) is related to location, but not identical. Carcinomas are epithelial cell cancers, sarcomas are connective tissue cancers, lymphomas are immune cell cancers, and so on. Different cancers respond best to different treatment options, so knowing what kind of cancer someone has is a critical first step.

I offer this incredibly simplified oncology primer to draw our attention to the challenges of cancer diagnosis. It's not just "cancer or not cancer?" but, rather, "which type of cancer?" This is a challenging question, but it is also a pressing question. Early diagnosis maximizes a cancer patient's chances of remission and recovery. The sooner you find a cancer, the sooner you can treat a cancer. This is all the more true if you can discover the cancer prior to significant tumor growth or metastasis. Many prospective cancer-screening regimes (think mammography awareness) were initially conceived based on this idea. (Although, more recent research indicates that the costs of these campaigns may outweigh the benefits.[14]) In most cases, diagnosing cancer is about looking at potential tumors. Mammography and X-rays can find clumps of cells that might be tumors, but the gold standard for diagnosis is a fine-needle aspirant (often called a biopsy). This is where doctors extract a small clump of suspicious cells and then use a microscope to examine them further.

Cancers look weird, and that's a good thing (sort of). Mutated, fast-growing cells can be identified early because they look different from normal healthy cells. But, at early stages cancer diagnosis is often part art and part science. "Normal" in a medical context is not uniform. Cells vary from tissue type to tissue type and from person to person. Even cancerous cells vary based on type and progression. Pathologists and oncologists have developed quantitization regimes to help minimize the ambiguity of diagnosis. Suspect cells are rated according to a range of categories that might indicate carcinogenesis. Thickness, uniformity, size, marginal adhesion, mitosis (cell division), and bare nuclei can all be assessed as part of diagnosis. With this kind of quantitization regime already in use, we have the ideal context for diagnostic AI development.

A study on algorithmic cancer diagnosis provides an ideal illustration of this kind of work.[15] The authors ground their study in the previously mentioned exigencies, namely, (1) the relatively high rates of breast cancer in the United States, and (2) the benefits of early detection. They further set up the need for their AI-driven approach by remarking on the challenges of common diagnostic methods:

> The commonly used diagnostic techniques, like mammography and fine needle aspiration cytology (FNAC), are reported to lack of [sic] high diagnostic capability. Therefore, there is an absolute necessity in developing better diagnostic techniques. Owing to the above-mentioned needs, expert systems and machine learning techniques are introduced to help improve the diagnostic capability.[16]

In reaching toward this goal, the authors offer a tour of each of the previously identified primary AI development processes. Through a review of the study's data curation, feature engineering, modeling, and benchmarking processes, the machinations of blackboxing engines become all the more apparent. Subsequently, in what follows, I address each development task in turn.

Data Curation

AI developers must acquire or curate a data set of previously evaluated cases taken to represent "ground truth" (see Chapter 4). This is essentially equivalent to the housetraining map in the opening to this chapter. Feature engineering is one of many processes that are designed to make the data more legible to computers. It's how you take whatever data you've got and make them into the kinds of numbers computers can read. Quantification and quantitization (see the Introduction) are the bread and butter of feature engineering. To stick with the housetraining example just a bit longer, one way to feature-engineer the data set might be to put my house and yard on a coordinate system. Then each pee place could be labeled based on its x- and y-axis positions. If my curb is at $y = 1$ and my front door is at $y = 5$, then an ML system could quickly learn that bad pee places typically start around $y > 5$. Data curation has, perhaps, received the most significant public attention as a risk vector for bias in AI. Insufficiently diverse and already biased data sets fuel bad AI. When inequity is already baked into the data, it's nearly impossible to develop a system that avoids replicating the inherent bias in the data.

In terms of the specific study I address in this chapter, it begins with a preexisting canonical data set of biopsy slides, the Wisconsin Breast Cancer Dataset (WBCD). This data set comes pre-engineered with grading data according to nine attributes describing cell shape, size, and distribution. Specific attributes included clump thickness, uniformity of cell size, uniformity of cell shape, marginal adhesion, single epithelia cell size, bare nuclei, gland chromatin, normal nucleoli, and mitoses. These are the things oncologists and pathologists are trained to look for. They are the visual features that doctors use when making a cancer diagnosis based on a biopsy. The grades are part of a quantitization regime based on perceived normalcy. So, a cell cluster with apparently normal distribution between cells would be graded as a 1 for clump thickness. In contrast, a slide with an exceptionally high rate of bare nuclei would be rated as a 10.

As a canonical data set, the WBCD is widely used in ML benchmarking. However, there is one striking limitation—the published data set includes no demographic data on patients. Age, race, ethnicity, and gender are all rendered invisible. In *Data Feminism*, D'Ignazio and Klein identify "privilege hazard" as a major driver of inequitable data sets. Privilege hazard occurs "when data teams are primarily composed of people from dominant groups [and], those perspectives come to exert outsized influences on the decisions being made—to the exclusion of inter identities and perspectives."[17] A common example of privilege hazard in tech is the predominantly white development team who put together a turn-by-turn GPS system that would tell users to "Turn right on Malcolm the Tenth Boulevard." Another increasingly pervasive example is accent bias in voice-activated technology. As Halycon Lawrence notes, digital assistants like Siri discipline users, forcing them to adopt a narrow range of accents in Standard American or Received British English in order to be heard and understood.[18] These glitches are classic examples of everyday casual racism, but privilege hazard often also leads to biased data sets with even more significant consequences for already marginalized communities. While missing demographic metadata might not seem like an issue for a data set on cell clumps, health disparities research indicates that there are significant differences in biopsy data and results by ethnicity.[19] As is typically the case, race-related differences are almost certainly the result of racialized inequity rather than any biological factor:

> Although race/ethnicity was also associated with biopsy results (Table 1), we do not interpret these data as necessarily reflecting lower biological risk among minority women. The quality of biopsies and pathology may be associated with socioeconomic status, and the completeness and accuracy of self-reported results may be associated with educational attainment, which was associated with race/ethnicity in our data (Table 1). Patients' socioeconomic status and race/ethnicity may also affect the quantity and quality of information that their physician provides about the need for or results of a biopsy.[20]

Now certainly, it is possible that appropriate demographic data are available somewhere, but I've got pretty good Google skills, and I can't find them. Most of the original citations for the WBCD are archived or offline entirely. Even if the data are somewhere obvious that I've missed, they are clearly not brought to bear in most studies that use the WBCD, including within the study in question. Since demographic data are not available for the WBCD, it is impossible to discern whether these issues compromise the integrity of the data; however, it is certainly plausible. Ultimately, the WBCD's status as a canonical data set allowed the data set itself to be blackboxed by citation. With a quick reference to a now-dead link, the research team moved on quickly to feature engineering and modeling.

Feature Engineering

Sometimes feature engineering is the most difficult part of AI development. As mentioned previously, it is a special challenge for AI that "reads" text and images. Transforming human language or photographs into numbers is no easy task. However, with respect to the current case, much of the work of feature engineering had been completed before the study. This is because WBCD essentially comes pre-engineered. The grade scores for each variable and each case were provided in advance. However, that doesn't mean there was no work to be done. AI is multiply expensive. It requires time, money, and computational resources and can have significant environmental impacts. If developers can identify a subset of features that are equally predictive of target outcomes (when compared with the whole set), they can save on these expenses. While specific issues like environmental costs were not identified as a driving exigency, the study behind "A Support Vector Machine Classifier with Rough Set-Based Feature Selection for Breast Cancer Diagnosis" was, nevertheless, centrally focused on reducing the costs of AI. As the title suggests, the underlying approach to breast cancer diagnosis in this paper combines the benefits of SVM (support vector machine) algorithms with "rough set-based feature selection."

Feature reduction or feature optimization is part of larger feature-engineering processes. The goal is to create a minimum viable "map" of the target phenomenon, so that the model can make accurate predictions at lower computational costs. Feature reduction often works in concert with modeling. Different feature batches, if you will, are submitted to modeling and compared through benchmarking. In terms of feature reduction in the current article, the authors use a mathematical approach called rough set (RS) theory. As they note,

> One of the major applications of RS theory is the attribute reduction that is the elimination of attributes. The reduction of attributes is achieved by comparing equivalence relations generated by sets of attributes. Using the dependency degree as a measure, attributes are

removed and reduced set provides the same dependency degree as the original.[21]

Essentially, the authors ran the same model seven times using seven different combinations of the nine available features. In the end, set #5 (Clump Thickness, Uniformity of Cell Shape, Marginal Adhesion, Bare Nuclei, Mitoses) showed the highest classification accuracy at 99.41%.[22]

The rough set approach, as deployed in this case, does not necessarily raise serious red flags in terms of bias. While data curation, feature engineering, modeling, and benchmarking all provide vectors for bias, those vectors are not necessarily active in every case of AI development. Nevertheless, feature engineering is often a major vector for bias in AI broadly and deep medicine specifically. Identified features do not always predict precisely what they are supposed to predict. This is the problem of proxies. The example of pulse oximetry from the Introduction is one of the most poignant examples of this. The double ratio of red to infrared light absorption is a proxy measure of oxygen saturation, but the relationship of that ratio to actual oxygen saturation is attenuated by skin color. Now it is possible to do equitable pulse oximetry based on light absorption. In fact, it was the industry standard several decades ago.[23] In the 1970s physicians would do a blood draw to set baseline oxygenation levels and then use the light absorption data to make inferences from those baseline levels. While proxies can be useful in deep medicine, it is critically important that selected proxies either reliably represent underlying features or that they are used in a context that corrects for the margin of error.

Modeling

Modeling is where things start to get a bit more complicated. In short, a model is a useful representation of an object, process, or data set. *Useful* is the key term here. Models are about making future tasks easier to accomplish more than they are about perfect accuracy. Think about the last time you changed a lightbulb. What did you do first? I hope it was turn off the switch. Maybe you are super safety minded and even turned off the breaker. You obviously don't want to get electrocuted. But let's take a minute to think about the thought process behind flipping the switch. On a basic level, you know having an open circuit is an electrocution hazard—one best avoided. You do not want power flowing through the broken lightbulb when you go to unscrew it. *Flowing*? That's an interesting word. Does electricity really flow? So, I am going to be honest with you here for a second. When I change a lightbulb or install a new fixture, I think about electricity like it is water. I imagine it *flowing* through pipes, and I dam up those pipes (flip the switch) at certain times to make sure I don't hurt myself. Sure—deep down—I know electricity is about electron transfer along conductive materials. But electrons don't really matter when I change a lightbulb. I don't need to think about orbital shells to get the job done. It's extraneous information.

Models like electricity-as-water are obviously incorrect, but they are also extremely useful. We use mental models all the time to filter out unneeded information and focus our attention on the job that needs to be done. Most of the time, mental models are helpful, but sometimes your default mental model gets in the way. Let's say I need to swap out a stick of RAM in my computer. Electricity-as-water isn't going to cut it. If I don't think about electricity in more sophisticated ways that involve static discharge, I might just fry my motherboard. The water model of electricity is the wrong model for this job. The statistical models that drive AI aren't quite the same as mental models, but the goals are the same. Again, from *Artificial Intelligence in Medicine*, "A model serves two main functions: (1) to predict the outcomes of future/unseen cases and (2) to provide insights into the underlying processes that contribute to the outcome of interest."[24] AI systems use algorithms to create statistical models that allow users to predict outcomes in future cases. The pre-classified training data, once feature engineered, are sorted and filtered through algorithms like k-nearest neighbor (KNN) or regression algorithms that make up SVMs. Specific algorithms or sets of algorithms are often what researchers are referring to when they use the term "architecture." AI models are built on underlying architectures (processes, procedures, statistical frameworks, etc.) that make prediction possible. Algorithms in architectures create statistical models that support future classification and prediction tasks. They essentially say, given a certain range of parameters (the engineered features), we can predict a certain outcome—e.g., for any given location in my yard or house (say x = 3, y = 2), we can predict its classification (good pee place). As mentioned above, SVM architectures deploy algorithms designed to identify the most efficient dividing line between classes. However, the toy model SVM represented in Figure 1.1 (right) hints at a linearity that is seldom possible. It imagines that you can draw a clean, straight line between classes. Very few data sets play nice like this. In fact, very few data sets can be appropriately modeled in two-dimensional space, and thus actual hyperplanes drawn by SVMs tend to look like geometers' nightmares. Even the silly thought experiment with housetraining my dog is a more true-to-life hyperplane.

The variables that drive model classifications are shaped by the statistical processes of machine learning. However, the process of modeling typically has to resolve conflicts in the data set. Even a six-dimensional plot of the relevant data will not really allow for an efficient and straight line. Thus, just like data curation and feature engineering, model selection and chosen tuning parameters can have a significant impact on the equity of AI systems. Models often automate the process of selecting or weighing features. Thus, the modeling process may select some features as more important for decision-making and in so doing minimize others. This offers a real possibility of increasing apparent accuracy at the expense of equity. An accurate modeling process makes reliable predictions based on the available data. But if that data or the features chosen to represent that data are marked by preexisting inequitable decision-making processes, then those inequitable processes will be learned by the model. However, even in the absence of such prior inequities (were such an absence possible), the way models manipulate and slice data, so to speak, can still produce favorable outcomes for some groups over others.

Benchmarking

And, finally, benchmarking tells us how good a trained model is at predicting the target outcome or classification. Benchmarking is so central to the process of AI development that Tom Mitchell, of the Machine Learning Department at Carnegie Mellon, even makes it part of the definition. As he writes, "we say that a machine *learns* with respect to a particular task T, performance metric P, and type of experience E, if the system reliably improves its performance P at task T, following experience E."[25] As we will see, that "metric P"[26] is a critical part of AI development and blackboxing. In fact, I will go so far as to argue that benchmarking metrics are the primary blackboxing engines of AI development. They are what allows researchers and developers to take a disarticulated system of humans, data, and architectures and transform them into an AI. Benchmarking is a critical part of closing the black box. As I will describe below, the act of assigning a score to a system in development is a critical component of what renders that system *a* system, and in so doing it occludes the development processes and vectors for potential bias.

The breast cancer detection AI system we are exploring in this chapter was trained on 683 labeled biopsy slides from the WBCD—444 classified as benign and 239 as malignant. Evaluating the effectiveness of AI systems is a somewhat complicated process. The above classification accuracy value (99.41%) is the easiest to calculate. It is a simple answer to the question: What percentage of the time did the AI get it right? In this case, if the AI was asked to evaluate 100 biopsy slides for malignancy, it would pick the right answer about 99 times. Classification accuracy is useful, but misleading. Write "malignant" on one side of a coin and "benign" on the other. Then flip that coin for biopsy. Statistically, you'll get about 50 correct diagnoses. Ninety-nine correct is still impressive, but maybe not so impressive if you are starting from 50. Another issue is that there are two ways to be wrong. A positive breast cancer finding is wrong if you do not have breast cancer. A negative finding is wrong if you do. Each of these situations is bad and can result in significant patient harm, but very different patient harm. Correcting for chance and differentiating between true positives, false positives, true negatives, and false negatives has become a cottage industry in data science and diagnostics. Classification accuracy, sensitivity, specificity, precision, recall, intraclass correlation coefficient, and area under the curve (AUC) comprise just a partial list of metrics designed to assess accuracy, validity, and/or agreement. Some of these metrics come from diagnostic medicine, others from data science, and still others from psychology. While different metrics are optimized for different use cases (about which, more in Chapter 4), it's not uncommon for AI developers to take the kitchen sink approach. While this particular study focuses primarily on classification accuracy, the authors offer specificity, sensitivity, and AUC scores along the way.

CLOSING THE BLACK BOX

Ultimately, this tour of AI development tells us a lot about blackboxing processes. The progression from data curation and feature engineering to modeling and benchmarking makes up the primary blackboxing engines in health AI. It is the story of how a collection of disparate parts and practices become an integrated thing. The blackboxing, itself, is forecasted in the article's introduction. As the authors write,

> In order to make great use of the advantages of RS theory in preprocessing the breast cancer data, and further improve the classification accuracy of the SVM predictor model, RS_SVM is proposed to diagnose the breast cancer in this work. This method consists of two-stages. In the first stage, RS is employed as an attribute reduction tool to extract the optimal features. This provides elimination of unnecessary data. In the second stage, the optimal feature subset is used as the inputs to a SVM classifier with good generalization performance.[27]

This passage essentially tells the whole story where RS and SVM are combined into a thing that is RS_SVM. For most of the outset of the article RS is a "theory," and SVM is a "theory" or a "concept." Even in the foreshadowing above RS_SVM is "a two-stage method." But in sections 4.4 and 4.5, everything changes, or, rather, RS_SVM changes into a thing. The first stage of thingification in this case comes when RS_SVM is granted its own "architecture."[28] The prior focus on processes and methods gives way to a metaphor of foundation and solidity. And, finally, once the benchmarking and assessments enter the frame, RS_SVM is fully a thing: "In order to evaluate the prediction performance of RS_SVM classifier, we define and compute the classification accuracy, sensitivity, specificity and ROC curves, respectively."[29] In this case, the simple conceit of the underscore illustrates blackboxing beautifully. The underscore that connects RS and SVM when combined with the attendant nominalization of *the* system is literally essential to how, as Latour puts it, the "many elements are made to act as one."[30]

As the collected research in critical algorithm studies amply demonstrates, the closing of the black box opens up new potential avenues for danger. When a system becomes a thing, questions about its inner workings recede into the background. A fully formed black box can be used, reused, deployed, and redeployed. Within deep medicine, a blackboxed health AI can be used in drug discovery, in clinical decision-making, and to support an everyday-healthy lifestyle. To be sure, all of these uses can lead to improvements in health, quality of care, and even, in some cases, equity. However, a black box not only holds technical details. It also holds trust. Because the black box of health AI is borne out of benchmarking, that benchmarking becomes the guarantee of trustworthiness. Benchmarking supports belief in system quality and utility without access to the inner machinations of that system. The benchmark-verified blackboxing allows clinicians, administrators, patients, and publics to defer to the guidance offered by blackboxed systems. In some cases, devotees of health AI treat those as digital oracles and follow maxims accordingly. There is obviously great risk here. Misplaced trust in AI has led to great harm in a wide variety of sectors. And deep medicine is no exception. Subsequently, in the next chapter, I explore in more detail how health AI can take on an oracular character and how trust in digital oracles can lead to dangerously misplaced surety.

Digital Oracles

Know thyself
Nothing to excess
Surety brings ruin

—Maxims of the Oracle at Delphi

These three maxims were etched into a column in the forecourt of the Temple of Apollo at Delphi (8th century BCE). The Temple is, of course, famous for being the place one went to see Pythia, the Oracle at Delphi. The Oracle is featured widely in ancient Greek writing from Herodotus, to Homer, to Plato and was revered as a sage and a guide. Her reputation was such that it was apparently common for those of means and wealth to endure significant pilgrimages to receive counsel. As a religious oracle, Pythia is shrouded in myth and mystery. Most accounts suggest that a visit to Pythia required participation in opaque rituals, possible exposure to hallucinogenic gases, and a willingness to trust in somewhat vague predictions. At this point, I will confess to a strong temptation to reread AI through the figure of Pythia. There's much in data curation, feature engineering, modeling, and expert systems recommendations that could be read as ritual, hallucinogen, and misplaced trust. However, for the most part I will avoid this figurative rereading and focus instead on the historical connection between the Oracle at Delphi and deep medicine—the god Apollo. In ancient Greek religion, Apollo was the god of archery, music, truth, prophecy, and medicine. The original Hippocratic oath begins with a pledge to Apollo, and it is no accident that Hippocrates argues that prognostics (foreknowing, foreseeing, and foretelling) should be the first art of medicine.

The Doctor and the Algorithm. S. Scott Graham, Oxford University Press. © Oxford University Press 2022.
DOI: 10.1093/oso/9780197644461.003.0003

More recently (since about 1796), diagnostics has been considered the first art of medicine. It has thus long been central for activating medicine's sociotechnical systems. A diagnosis authorizes. It activates potential treatment plans. It justifies the use of specific medicines. Its corresponding billing code even makes payment available for insured patients. However, with the increasing availability of new technologies for predictive modeling (including AI), prognosis has begun to return to center stage in medicine's sociotechnical systems. This renewed oracular mode of medicine also coincides with increasing investments in preventative, precision, and personalized medicine. You generally do not visit an oracle for insights about the broad course of history. You visit an oracle to find out what is going to happen to *you*. Likewise, any of the central promises of deep medicine revolve around their purported ability to make personalized predictions about your individual future health. These new digital oracles will not tell you if you should flee the Spartans or if anyone is wiser than Socrates but, rather, if you should eat more kale or what your ideal sleep schedule might be. Armed with these custom-tailored predictions, the hope is that you can stave off illness and death for, at least, a few more years.

For the most part, the oracular mode of medicine follows directly from hype in health AI. That is, the overly expansive promises about AI's future and what AI can do for your future are less about individual technologies currently in development and more a result of futurism. In the Introduction to this book, I described this oracular turn as an attempt to remake medicine anew. However, as mentioned above, this idea that oracular medicine is medicine made anew is only partially true. The parallels between our new digital oracles and the ancient Hippocratic approach to medicine are more than surface level. So, in what follows, I will explore a very brief history of Western medicine in terms of the shift from prognostics to diagnostics and back again. Using this history as a foundation, I will then outline how the new digital oracles of deep medicine embody the first two maxims of the Delphic oracle: (1) know thyself and (2) nothing to excess. And, finally, this chapter will close with a consideration of the last maxim. Specifically,

I argue that a certain strain of technochauvinism leads to a deep and misplaced trust in deep medicine. This surety has already brought ruin in other AI sectors, and it is a significant threat to the real potential benefits of health AI.

THERE AND BACK AGAIN: THE FIRST ART OF WESTERN MEDICINE

Western medicine has been historically centered around four primary activities: diagnosis, prognosis, treatment, and prevention. Over the course of medical history, different eras have anointed different "firsts among equals" from among these four activities. For Hippocrates, prognosis was the first discipline of medicine. Importantly, this ancient approach to prognosis was significantly inflected by cultural investments in the god Apollo. Hippocrates' *Book of Prognostics* was one of the most important works in what has become known as the Hippocratic Corpus, and it begins by championing the importance of prediction:

> It appears to me a most excellent thing for the physician to cultivate Prognosis; for by foreseeing and foretelling, in the presence of the sick, the present, the past, and the future, and explaining the omissions which patients have been guilty of, he will be the more readily believed to be acquainted with the circumstances of the sick; so that men will have confidence to entrust themselves to such a physician.[1]

This focus on prognosis makes a lot of sense in a context where treatment options were rather rudimentary when compared with today's standards. Being able to tell a patient how a condition would progress was a central part of a clinical practice where cures were hard to come by. Interestingly, Hippocrates links prognosis directly to clinical trust. When curative options are meager, the ability to predict the course of a disease may well be the best way to demonstrate expertise and foster trust.

Over the centuries, as more effective treatment options became available, prognosis has become less central to Western medicine.[2] The decline of prognostics began in the 18th century and coincided with the slow emergence of diagnosis as medicine's new first art. As the germ theory of disease began to displace Hippocratic, Galenic, and miasmic medicine, clinical attention shifted away from prediction in two stages: first, a reorientation toward preventative medicine, and second, a subsequent valorization of diagnosis as medicine's first art. In the U.S. context, the preventative century is bookended by two major historic developments in public health. The first laws requiring smallpox quarantine and isolation were passed in Massachusetts in 1701,[3] and Edward Jenner developed the smallpox vaccine in 1796.[4] The mid-19th century marked the ascendency of diagnostic medicine with the pathology paradigm revolution ushered in by Rudolf Virchow.[5] Virchow is most famous for the microscopic identification of syphilis. By marshaling new technologies to identify specific illnesses, medicine could now offer a powerful new framework for clinical intervention. It is not uncommon for contemporary physicians to draw a more-or-less straight line between the development of microscopy and recent developments like PET scans and fMRI.[6]

Importantly, the shift from prognosis to diagnosis catalyzed a transformation of the dominant logics and networks of medicine. No longer was "foreseeing and foretelling" central. Rather, the new first art of medicine focused on the proper logical methods for identifying the true cause of illness based on sets of identified symptoms. The following passage from Barclay's 1862 *A Manual of Medical Diagnosis* is illustrative of the era:

All true diagnosis is ultimately based upon inductions separately framed out of clinical and pathological investigations and experiments. By careful and repeated observation, we have succeeded, with every appearance of truth, in associating certain phenomena observed during life with particular lesions found after death; and these form the first step in our progress. . . . In so far as we are able to correctly interpret symptoms, and to trace out in connection with them a real change of structure or of function which affords an adequate explanation of their presence, in so far are we prepared to form a correct diagnosis.[7]

With the final ascendence of diagnostics, the inductive inference replaces prognostic foresight as the dominant logic of medicine. While diagnostics would continue to be the uncontested first art for about another hundred years,[8] the underlying logics of diagnosis shifted with subsequent innovations in mathematics (particularly statistics) and thus paved the way for an eventual return of prognostic medicine.

There are many places one could look for possible "origin points" in statistical medicine. Eugenicists like Francis Galton and Karl Pearson certainly had significant impacts on its emergence. However, rather than focus on identifying some essential first moment, I will briefly turn to the text that revolutionized diagnostics—Jacob Yerushalmy's 1942 "Statistical Problems in Assessing Methods of Medical Diagnosis, with Special Reference to X-Ray Techniques."[9] Yerushalmy's article is most famous for introducing the concepts of and calculations for sensitivity and specificity. The overall article is motivated by his concern that there is no standard method for determining which among several different X-ray techniques leads to the most accurate diagnoses. Along the way, Yerushalmy rejects induction as an appropriate logical foundation for diagnosis and argues, instead, that all diagnosis is inherently probabilistic:

The process of medical diagnosis involves the application to a specific case of the knowledge accumulated from a large number of similar cases. This knowledge may have been derived by systematic observation and detailed analysis of case records, or it may have been obtained intuitively in the course of the physician's experience. In either instance the process is statistical in nature in that it consists of abstracting from a multiplicity of factors and conditions those which are pertinent to specific cases. Moreover, since no two cases are exactly alike, the resulting diagnoses are not absolute but involve some uncertainty and might better be thought of in terms of probabilities.[10]

While the article makes no overt reference to prediction, the recentering of diagnosis as probabilistic and statistical leads medicine rather quickly into predictive territory. When sensitivity and specificity are individualized, that is, used to evaluate the likelihood that a given patient will have a given illness based on the results of a given diagnostic test, positive predictive value (PPV) and negative predictive value (NPV) become the metrics of central importance.[11] As I have argued previously within the rubrics of the new statistical era of medicine, "Diagnostics is now a process of comparing the observed (or experimentally derived) signs and symptoms with statistical tables that help the clinician determine the additive probability of each new symptom."[12]

This quick tour from ancient prognoses to statistical diagnosis is a very rough sketch of the history of Western medicine. I would direct you to the many books by actual historians of medicine who would offer you a more sophisticated understanding of this history. However, this thumbnail sketch is sufficient to understand the context of AI in the broader milieu of contemporary Western medicine. Like the technological shifts that recentered medicine on diagnosis or prevention, devotees of AI offer the technology up as another profound recentering of medical science and clinical practice. In one sense this might be true. One thing that is perhaps unique about AI in the history of medicine is the way it collapses the long-standing divisions between the four practices of medicine. At its core, AI is a predictive technology. It makes probabilistic assessments given certain data and parameters. In some respects, this might recenter medicine back in a prognostic idiom. Historically, diagnosis was about hypothesis generation and even intuitive leaps. However, for the past 50 years, probabilistic reasoning has become increasingly important to diagnostic practices. Ultimately, the shift to predictive statistics has paved the way for a new, less mystic foundation, for prognosis.[13] AI extends and reifies these already ongoing transformations.

It is no accident that "PREDICT, PREDICT, PREDICT"[14] (literally three times in a row and in all caps) is a chapter subheading in Topol's *Deep Medicine*. AI is offered to the world broadly and to medicine specifically as an essentially predictive technology. In hospital settings especially, there is great enthusiasm for what predictive analytics might do to improve patient care. There are many new technologies under active development that aim to predict clinical outcomes (disease onset, disease progression) or health system usage (hospital readmission, transfer to intensive care). Broadly, developers hope that these technologies will more effectively guide and allocate care to improve health outcomes and/or reduce the costs of care. There are countless examples of new in-hospital prediction systems. Mostly they attempt to leverage electronic health records data to predict patient needs or outcomes. However, one of my favorite recent examples in this area uses a nurse "Worry Factor"[15] to predict intensive care transfers.

Specifically, the goal of Romero-Brufau et al.'s paper was to develop an AI system that might predict when hospitalized patients would deteriorate rapidly over a 24-hour period. As they note, "Detecting when a patient is deteriorating is critical to hospital care."[16] Deterioration can lead to "increased mortality if interventions are delayed."[17] Most in-hospital AI systems leverage electronic health records (EHRs). In an in-patient setting, this seems ideal. Vital signs are routinely monitored, and thus there may be a real chance of predicting deterioration based on this regularly updated data. Recognizing that the available literature on records-based prediction shows both low model validity and limited improvements in health outcomes, Romero-Brufau and his coauthors decided to try something new. They sought to capture the expert judgments of those in most regular contact with patients—nurses. Specifically, the goal was to evaluate "the predictive accuracy of nurses' judgment of risk, whether based on analytical or intuitive pattern recognition processes."[18] The study authors quantified nurse worry through a Worry Factor scale and supplied Worry Factor data to the model to test predictive accuracy. Impressively, quantitized nurse judgments were able to predict accurately 77% of patient deterioration events in the study. Even more impressively, models trained on nurse Worry Factor result in higher accuracy scores than most published AI early warning systems that rely on EHR data.[19]

Over the last fifty years, there have been several attempts to re-center prognosis in medicine.[20] These efforts have been stymied by a lack of predictive accuracy, a general reticence on the part of physicians to make prognostic judgments, and discomfort with notions like foreseeing and foretelling.[21] Enter AI. Quantitizing epistemologically suspect concepts like "worry" provides a more comfortable framework for clinicians in the era of evidence-based medicine. The increasing accuracy of AI systems may well lead to increased trust in prognostic predictions. With this increased acceptance and trust possibly on the horizon, some in deep medicine now advocate for revolutionary new approaches to personalized prognostic medicine. The previously discussed hospital predictive systems seem almost quaint compared with the grand visions of health AI techno-futurists. Thus, in what follows, I explore some of the more extravagant recommendations for digital oracles.

KNOW THYSELF

Atkins, South Beach, Glycemic Index, Whole Thirty, Intermittent Fasting—every year or so there is a new fad diet that promises to revolutionize your health and well-being. The diet industry is precisely that—an industry, and it is incredibly difficult to separate out the best scientific recommendations from baseless marketing. Part of this comes from the fact that nutrition science is notoriously difficult. Topol argues that "Most nutrition science is predicated on observational and retrospectively gathered data, which is dependent on people accurately reporting what they eat. 'Accurately reporting' could be thought of as an oxymoron."[22] And while I will not be as critical of retrospective and reporting-based data as he is, variable control and good data are extremely difficult to come by. The nutrition science with the most rigorously collected data comes from studies that lock participants in controlled settings to be fed and monitored by researchers—not something that will ever approximate real eating habits. Nutrition science is also notorious for its financial conflicts of interest.[23] I used to teach in a food science building, and I will never forget walking by the display case of prestigious awards won by members of the nutrition faculty. One of those awards was provided by the Pringles corporation to celebrate a faculty member's unique contributions to fry oil. The award was a custom can of Pringles snack chips, and each chip had a color photo of the scientist printed on its surface. In addition to these challenges to nutrition science, there is an increasing recognition that there is no such thing as "The Best Diet" but, rather, "*your* best diet." As Topol argues,

> This indeed is the biggest problem facing nutrition guidelines— the idea that there is simply one diet that all human beings should follow. The idea is both biologically and physiologically implausible, contradicting our uniqueness, the remarkable heterogeneity and individuality of our metabolism, microbiome, environment, to name a few dimensions.[24]

Compelling evidence supports these claims, and AI is presented as the ideal guide to help us identify the best diet for us. As Topol puts it, "To transcend the evidence-free universal diet concept, it takes a computational, data-driven unbiased approach."[25]

In the new era of medical digital oracles, knowing thyself is critical to identifying the best approaches for your unique individual health. In the context of diet recommendations systems, this means feeding the system copious amounts of data, so that the system can better feed you. Per Topol, "Getting all of a person's data amalgamated is the critical first step."[26] In anchoring these claims, Topol turns to a 2015 *Cell* article on "Personalized Nutrition by Prediction of Glycemic Responses."[27] The study details the creation of a personalized food recommendation system, built on predictions of your personalized glycemic response, essentially blood sugar and glucose levels. The paper is built on the idea that individual glycemic response can be highly predictive of food metabolization. Through attenuating your diet to your glycemic response, you can (in theory) maintain a target weight. The glycemic response prediction system collected data on gut microbiota, blood chemistry, anthropometrics, sleep, exercise, and eating habits for eight hundred participants, aged 18–70.[28] Ultimately, the researchers were able to build a model that reliably predicted glycemic response within the contexts of the study. These data were ultimately leveraged to make targeted diet recommendations for each individual. While fascinating, this research is not without its criticism. An editorial run in the *European Journal of Clinical Nutrition* shortly after the original publication criticizes this glycemic-index-based digital oracle as pure "fantasy."[29] The author criticizes the original study for many of the common failings of AI. Specifically, he cites a "flawed rationale"[30] and "irrelevant" surrogate endpoints.[31] A 2018 *Gut* meta-study of this and other approaches to AI-driven diet advice criticizes the field broadly for showing a lack of compelling clinical evidence:

> Although found as highly promising and clearly showing the application by some researchers, others have requested to tone down the potentiality of a broad applicability with conclusions such as the fact that predictive algorithms are black boxes with complex statistical associations without the real mechanisms explaining the presence of such associations. Or others mentioned that the results do not provide enough evidence that the model is finally superior to the current methods of detecting high glucose levels and even did not demonstrate that personalised nutrition advice are superior to standard advice in view of managing high glucose levels in postprandial situations.[32]

Recognizing the limitations of early efforts, researchers Hamideh, Arellano, Topol (same one), and Steinhubl call for more and increasingly rigorous research into digital nutritionists.[33] Nevertheless, while the scientific jury is largely still out on the question of AI-guided personalized nutrition, that has not stopped algorithmic personal nutrition from entering the marketplace.

At the time of this writing, intermittent fasting is perhaps the most in-vogue diet plan, and recent months have seen a flurry of new putatively AI-based smartphone apps that promise to help you calibrate your nutritional needs and fasting schedule to your own unique physiology.[34] Given the broad challenges to effective nutrition research, questionable model data, and regular concerns about the purported mechanisms of actions that underwrite the latest dieting innovations, it remains to be seen whether diet-related digital oracles will effectively provide the touted benefits. Nevertheless, their presence and increasing popularization signals a significant shift in clinical logics. Advocates of health AI seek to usher in a new oracular era of medicine grounded in precision recommendations tailored to individual physiologies. What's more, the most strident proponents of health AI hope that this new oracular era will be marked by 24/7 monitoring and continuous targeted lifestyle arguments. Thus, deep medicine tacitly invokes the Oracle at Delphi's second maxim (nothing to excess).

NOTHING TO EXCESS

According to many personal–health system advocates, the true promise of personalized predictive health AI simply cannot be realized without a constant stream of high-quality data. As Topol argues, the best health AI systems will have "to be nurtured, fed with all the new and relevant data, be they from a sensor, life stress event, a change in career path, results of a gut microbiome test, birth of a child and on and on."[35] An entire life subject to ongoing quantification and quantitization—you must be processed, analyzed, aggregated, and sorted so that your data can be transformed into actionable recommendations offered up at the ideal moment for intervention. In short, the sociotechnical networks of deep medicine should surround all aspects of your daily life. Concrete proposals build on ideas like those expressed by Topol and argue for whole suites of sensors that will measure vital signs, record activity, track location, monitor social media, administer on-demand blood tests, and take targeted mental health inventories.

Jaeho et al.'s chapter in *Artificial Intelligence in Medicine* describes the creation of just such a system. See Figure 2.1 for a model that integrates monitoring of diet, fitness and physical activity, sleep, sexual/reproductive health, and mental health. As the authors detail, these manifold data will

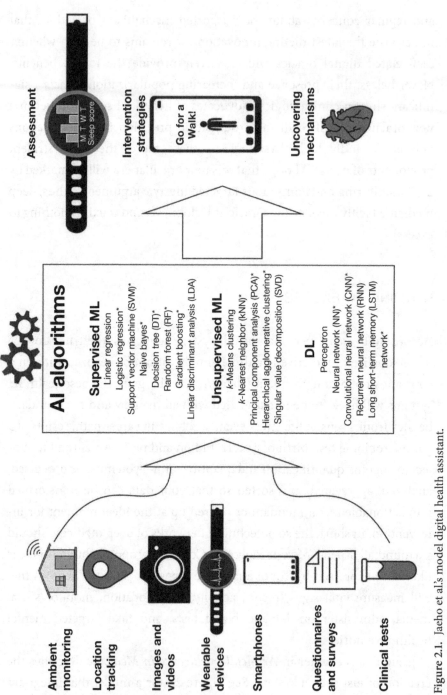

Figure 2.1. Jaeho et al.'s model digital health assistant. Adapted from Jaeho et al.

be sifted and sorted by various supervised and unsupervised AI systems and transformed into quantitized measures that can inform your daily life (e.g., a sleep score) or specific recommendations ("take a walk"). There's much excitement about these sorts of "just-in-time adaptive interventions" or JITAIs. As a recent National Academy of Medicine report on the future of health AI notes,

> The JITAI makes decisions about when and how to intervene based on response to prior intervention, as well as on awareness of current context, whether internal (mood, anxiety, blood pressure), or external (e.g., location, activity). JITAI assistance is provided when users are most in need of it or will be most receptive to it.[36]

For Jaeho et al., the overarching justification for all-pervasive JITAI is current population-level mortality data. Specifically, the authors cite "non-communicable chronic diseases" like heart disease, obesity, and stress-related conditions as the primary global drivers of illness and death.[37] Subsequently, they argue that a digital health assistant is a critical intervention because these common causes of death "result mainly from unhealthy behaviors and can be prevented by adopting healthier lifestyles."[38] Jaeho et al's proposed system is vaporware. It is a concept paper. But real digital health assistants are currently available for purchase and subscription. Vessel's in-home wellness tracker, for example, offers an integrated smartphone app and daily urinalysis test kit that purportedly can be used to improve your health through targeted recommendations.[39] Vessel recommendations combine AI-driven advice on exercise, diet, and weight management with available in-app purchases for custom vitamins, the formulation of which appears to be based on your daily in-home urinalysis findings.

The overarching health behavior foundation of these real and imaginary systems is the primary reason I address 24/7 monitoring digital health assistants under the rubric of "nothing to excess." These apps and AIs largely embody an outdated vision of moderation- and temperance-based health. Indeed, they connect directly to Hippocrates' opening lines and his articulation of the clinical duty to explain "the omissions which patients have been guilty of." Although Jaeho et al.'s article makes a quick reference to social determinants of health (SDoH), the very idea of JITAI centers behavioral interventions as the primary mode of intervention for health. While there can be reasonable disagreements about the relative contribution of social, genetic, and behavioral determinants, medicine has historically vastly underestimated SDoH at a huge cost to health equity.[40] A personalized oracular model of deep medicine, as exemplified by the digital health assistant, ultimately reifies the behavioral approach. While data on socioeconomic status, race, ethnicity, and so on might populate these decision systems, individualized recommendations will never address the root causes of health injustice. Even if an app alert did suggest something more appropriate to SDoH like "join a health equity coalition and vote for candidates who support socialized medicine," that kind of alert obviously is not going to tear down the walls of inequitable access to care or voting booths for that matter.

SURETY BRINGS RUIN

The "problem" of trust in AI is now a common issue of concern across AI sectors. Technologists and AI advocates regularly lament that users, communities, and governments do not trust algorithmic technologies. But the foundational assumption that AI is not trusted is not necessarily warranted. As a survey conducted by the Oxford University Center for Governance of AI found that a slim majority (51%) of Americans, for example, support AI development.[41] Importantly, however, they also found that those who support AI the most tend to be "wealthy, educated, male, or have experience with technology."[42] Certainly many do not trust AI, and those wo don't are, quite understandably, those who are at the greatest risk of being adversely affected by inequitable AI. So, if we have a situation where wealthy, educated, male technologists already trust a product, and marginalized groups do not, the problem of "trust" starts to look a bit like a marketing gimmick. Importantly, somewhere along the way the idea of trust in AI came to overshadow the goal of making trustworthy AI. Trust is a poor surrogate measure for the quality of a system, with significant potential detriments. As a recent *Journal of Medical Internet Research* article notes,

> It is also important to note that maximizing the user's trust does not necessarily yield the best decisions from a human-AI collaboration. When trust is at maximum, the user accepts or believes all the recommendations and outcomes generated by the AI system. While in some applications, AI can outperform human decision-making by incorporating data from multiple sources, the limitations above suggest that unnecessarily high trust in AI may have catastrophic consequences, especially in life-critical applications.[43]

Importantly, this is not just idle speculation. Recent research has found that a focus on AI trust can lead to significant problems. When the focus is trust rather than trustworthiness, recommended solutions focus on interventions like explainability. As the basic logic goes, AIs are a black box, and so if we better understand them, we will trust them. Subsequently, recent years have seen significant emphasis on eXplainable AI (XAI) systems. XAI tools highlight the parameters most likely to influence model recommendations. They visualize and simplify algorithmic results to make predictions more intuitive to human users, thereby fostering trust.

As mentioned above, there is some evidence to suggest that AI systems that prioritize explainability and interpretability may result in unintended pernicious effects. A recent study of XAI decision aids found that users were more likely to defer unreflectively to algorithmic judgments when they could more readily understand the foundations of the AI's predictions.[44] Critically, this deference to the algorithm persisted even when the predictions made were wildly off base. Counterintuitively, it may be that the critical posture encouraged by a more opaque system results in better overall decision-making. Similar studies have found that XAI decision aids can increase user confidence in their own AI-informed judgments (in clinical and nonclinical settings) without increasing the accuracy of those judgments.[45] These results persist even in cases where users are highly trained domain area experts and therefore raise serious concerns about suggestions that human intervention can blunt the worst excesses of AI.[46] Studies of AI-generated diet advice have also found that XAI significantly increases user trust in recommendations, even when those explanations are intentionally false.[47] Ultimately, XAI and other trust-bolstering decisions have the practical effect of making users more confident in AI recommendations. But *users* are often not even those most affected by AI decisions. In health AI contexts, the focus primarily has been on fostering increased clinician trust. Indeed, it is not necessarily assumed that patients will even know that AI systems are involved in clinical decision-making. Up to 70% of doctors report using Wikipedia as part of clinical decision-making,[48] but I've certainly never had a doctor inform me of that fact. When it comes to AI, *STAT* reports that hospitals are generally "operating under the assumption that you do not disclose."[49] Increasing clinical trust without increasing AI trustworthiness or even patient awareness strikes me as an exemplar case of "surety brings ruin."

Critical algorithm studies has tackled the problem of misplaced surety before—although not always through the lens of "trust," per se. Broussard's analysis of the dangers of technochauvinism is especially instructive here. As she writes, "technochauvinism is the belief that tech is always the solution."[50] Specifically, this belief is driven by "the notion that computers are more 'objective' or 'unbiased' because they distill questions and answers down to mathematical evaluation"[51] and leads to "unwavering faith that if the world just used more computers, and used them properly, social problems would disappear and we'd create a new digital utopia."[52] Technochauvinism is an excellent way of identifying the root cause of misplaced trust. Broussard's analysis effectively captures the cultural conditions that lead to surety in AI systems, and she artfully traces that surety to all manner of ruin. Broussard is, of course, not alone. AI rhetorics of "overcoming bias" have been linked to undue trust across critical algorithm studies, and that perceived lack of bias has been traced to employment discrimination,[53] racist recidivism prediction,[54] and misogynistic search engine results.[55] Much of this research has focused on the pernicious results of systemic racism, occluded motivations, and even the inadvertent results of privilege hazard. As I close my discussion on undue trust in health AI, I will focus on some of the striking (and even shocking) things that AI advocates say out loud. To be clear, here I identify several moments where technochauvinism bubbles up to the surface in concerning ways. Technochauvinism is often subtle and subtextual. While moments as blunt as the examples that follow are usually rare in mainstream discourse, their presence is indictive of what lurks under the surface and thus represents cause for concern.

Clearly, misplaced surety in AI technologies can cause developers to overlook likely consequences of their new systems. This has been routinely shown to be a problem given the relatively homogeneous demographics of the tech industry. Privilege hazard prevents developers from seeing repercussions that would be obvious to more diverse teams. However, misplaced trust in AI systems also leads some to hand-wave away or even embrace recognized repercussions. For example, medical futurist Berci Meskó recently tweeted,

> No doubt: there's no #digitalhealth without sacrificing a part of our #privacy. It's not a question anymore whether we should do this, but how we can do it in a way that protects what is valuable and vulnerable.[56]

Here, it is not that he is unaware of the privacy ramifications related to 24/7 biometric and ambient monitoring. Rather, he has decided that the trade-offs are worth the cost because of the trust he places in the recommendations of these systems. Similarly, Topol's reflection on an apparent Chinese lead in the "AI arms race" comes with a startling valorization of state-sponsored mass surveillance:

> But it's China that seems positioned to take the lead in AI for medicine. So many important factors line up: unparalleled quantity of data collection (citizens cannot opt out of data collection), major

government and venture fund investment, major AI programs at most of the big universities, and a very supportive regulatory environment.[57]

Here again, it is not lack of awareness that is the issue. Rather, it is misplaced surety leading to an odd lament about the United States's comparatively more modest surveillance state.

Unfortunately, this is not a unique oversight. In several instances, *Deep Medicine* is quick to embrace problematic tech fixes as it advocates for an expansive vision of health AI. Topol celebrates the potential for Weibo- and Facebook-integrated mental health surveillance.[58] While large swaths of *Deep Medicine* are devoted to assuring doctors that they will still be needed in the era of health AI, he is all too willing to offer up nurses as a cost-saving measure:

> But AI could ultimately reduce the need for nurses, both in hospitals and in outpatient clinicals and medical offices. Using AI algorithms to process data from the remote monitoring of patients at home will mean that there is a dramatically reduced role for hospitals to simply observe patients, either to collect data or to see whether symptoms get worse or reappear.[59]

Perhaps Topol's trust in AI will lead to more trust in nurses given their critical importance to ICU admission prediction. Regardless, none of this can really be attributed to a lack of awareness. The fifth chapter of *Deep Medicine*, "Deep Liabilities," explores the many negative externalities associated with undue surety in AI. He invokes *Weapons of Math Destruction*, the best recommendations of the AI Now Institute, and critical reporting from *ProPublica*, demonstrating full awareness of AI's many failings. In the context of privacy and surveillance, Topol broadly recognizes the potential perils but offers up the tech fix of health data ownership as a panacea: "If you owned and controlled it, you'd have a far better chance of preventing theft, hacking, and selling of your data without your knowledge."[60] While I have some obvious concerns about *Deep Medicine*, it's important to note that Topol's recent publications have been more cautious. In fact, as I'll describe in Chapter 7, he's become an important voice in calls for more rigorous approaches to vetting the quality of health AI.

In some areas of health AI, the extent of technochauvinism can be downright shocking. In *Machine Learning and AI for Healthcare*, Arjun Panesar argues horrifyingly that "freedom of choice, and consent is ultimately a utopian concept."[61] He goes so far as to suggest that respecting user preferences about data privacy "is neither realistic nor plausible."[62] This argument is warranted by the odd claim that clinicians have a moral duty to violate patient preferences if their actions might prevent loss of life.[63] Obviously these arguments are entirely out of step with commonly accepted clinical practices and the core dictates of bioethics. In a classic case of technochauvism, Panesar dives headlong into making claims about healthcare and biomedical ethics despite being educated exclusively in mechanical engineering and computer science. And, certainly, a dedicated health technologist can learn enough about medicine and bioethics to make meaningful contributions to these areas, but that does not appear to have happened here. Later in the book, Panesar instructs readers that AI failures are often the result of human biases.[64] In so doing, he tells the story of Tay, Microsoft's AI chatbot who was trained by Internet trolls to parrot racist and sexist invective. This is an important cautionary tale about the dangers of AI. Yet, the takeaway message in *Machine Learning and AI for Healthcare* is that we should remove people from the equation so as to have efficient and ethical machines. As Panesar writes, "as long as humans are involved in decisions, a bias will always exist."[65] A few pages later, in a section entitled "Is Bias a Bad Thing?," Panesar argues that what appears to be evidence of bias in AI might be better understood as instructive about the true conditions of the world. This claim leads somehow to the argument that such realizations are "the beginning of a societal and philosophical conflict between two species."[66] I'm not entirely sure how such unflinching faith in technology's promises can be maintained in the face of a simultaneous belief that a human–AI conflict is on the horizon. This is the odd power of technochauvinism. Obviously, there are many people in the world who hold problematic and ill-considered views about technology. We don't have to confront every questionable viewpoint. But given that *Machine Learning and AI for Healthcare* was published by a division of Springer-Nature and written by a recipient of the U.K. National Health Service Innovation Accelerator fellowship, I think we have to address these arguments as a serious and deeply problematic part of health AI discourse.

Ultimately, the supreme confidence in AI and the deep medicine revolution to come is fueling unprecedented investments in Health AI. The promise of oracular technologies has led to a significant uptick in venture capital investments in this area. $4.7 billion in U.S. venture capital in 2015 was $14 billion by 2020.[67] This upward trend shows no sign of slowing and should represent a huge cause for concern. Many of the most promising advancements in deep medicine have been incubated in university hospitals and are the result of federal research funding. Hype-fueled venture capital tends to embrace the worst excesses of disruptive innovation (see Chapter 3) and is more likely to support misplaced surety in the putative benefits of new technology. Venture capital investments in private AI development have been largely responsible for the worst excesses of AI outside of healthcare. Unbridled enthusiasm for the digital oracles may well lead health AI to a very dark place, one built on a blithe acceptance of digital surveillance and a rejection of user rights. Melinda Cooper's *Life as Surplus* warns that a sort of "capitalist delirium" is already leading us to this dark place in biotech broadly.[68] As she argues, biotechnology under the auspices of capitalism run amok is "designed to relocate economic production at the genetic, microbial, and cellular level, so that life becomes, literally, annexed within capitalist processes of accumulation."[69]

CONCLUSION

Ultimately, the oracular orientation of AI and the re-embrace of prognostics have the potential to improve clinical care. If new technological systems can reliably predict patient outcomes, then we have a better chance of bringing the right interventions to bear at the right time. In this respect, hospital-based expert decision systems offer the most promising immediate future. If these systems can be built on the right model data (which often includes unduly neglected sources of information like SDoH data and expert nurse judgments), then we have a chance at trustworthy prognostic AI. "Trustworthy" is the key here, because, as this chapter has shown, trusted AI is often not trustworthy AI. Surety in predictions and unflinching belief in the tech fix has and will continue to lead to all manner of harms from health inequity to possibly even patient death. Currently the dangers of misplaced trust in health AI can be best seen through the unreflective embrace of personalized digital oracles. At present, digital health assistants built on dubious models and fed 24/7 surveillance data are more likely to contribute to your datafication than your health.

These digital oracles celebrate app culture and reify an antiquated notion of behavioral health. In-app vitamin purchases based on urinalysis and putatively algorithmic diet recommendations fold seamlessly into the logics of predatory capitalism. By individualizing health as a matter of personal decision-making and behavior, these tech fixes provide a steady stream of product-based solutions and distract attention from SDoH.[70] Health system access, environmental injustice, and racism in medicine are entirely unaddressed issues under the oracular framework, despite being well established as significant SDoH. This, combined with the willing embrace of surveillance technologies and social-media-integrated health solutions, offers a damning vision of huge swaths of health AI.

So, the most pressing question for deep medicine becomes about how to prioritize development that avoids the worst excesses of misplaced surety. As mentioned previously, I remain confident that AI already has and will continue to result in positive improvements in health and medicine. Encouraging those more positive pathways will require a more comprehensive understanding of how health AI is rendered oracular and invested with so much misplaced trust. Blackboxing is a key element in this equation. And, as noted in Chapter 1, blackboxing is a team sport. It requires the concerted and enduring efforts of communities of practice who continue to maintain the black box through its simultaneous use and deferral. This is a primary feature of making an AI but also of an AI making it. In

Chapter 1, I focused primarily on the first sense of making—the literal processes of fabrication through the engines of blackboxing. Data curation, feature engineering/optimization, modeling, and benchmarking are critical to the processes of blackboxing. But so, too, is the other sense of *make*—as in making it (as in "I've made it. I've finally made it.") A recurrent through line of *The Doctor and the Algorithm* is that making an AI is part and parcel to an AI making it. If a research team makes the best AI in history but no one uses it, it doesn't matter. Promotion (or dissemination to be less critical about it) is an essential aspect of health AI, one that begins at the earliest stages of conceptualization, alongside (if not before) actual development activities. As Latour notes, a black box has only truly arrived when it becomes portable, when the subsystems cohere and are occluded such that the new nominalized system can be taken up by others. As he describes it, "The black box moves in space and becomes durable in time only through the actions of many people . . . "[71]

Research reports, whether they take the form of scholarly articles or industry white papers, are thus one of the primary engines of black box portability. They serve to package up the new technology such that it can be taken up by new and larger systems. Those systems, if they maintain the black box, also contribute to enduring portability. They maintain the sense of closure around the thingified box. Such systems include regulatory agencies, professional medical associations, marketing, promotional initiatives, and so forth. To understand blackboxing is also to understand the portability of black boxes. And, so, in the next chapter it is precisely to this notion of an AI making it, to this idea of portability, that I must turn.

How to Make It as an AI

Scurvy is a serious medical condition. This sentence might strike you as odd if you are not well acquainted with the Age of Sail or the adverse health effects of extreme poverty or living unhoused. You might know that scurvy is the result of vitamin C deficiency but are perhaps less familiar with the signs and symptoms: fatigue, soreness, weakness, open sores, ulceration, bleeding gums. In that aforementioned Age of Sail (roughly 1571–1862), "shipowners and governments assumed a 50% death rate from scurvy for their sailors on any major voyage."[1] Famously, James Lind, a Scottish surgeon in the British Royal Navy, discovered that citrus fruit could be used to treat and prevent the condition in 1753. Those among my readers familiar with research on dissemination of science and innovation will recognize this story as a canonical tale of delayed innovation adoption. It has been a staple of the literature since, at least, Everett Rogers' germinal *Diffusion of Innovations*,[2] the first edition of which was published in 1962. As the story goes, despite Lind's profound clinical insight, it would be another 40 years before the British Royal Navy implemented a policy of providing lemon juice to sailors at the direction of physician Gilbert Blaine, the newly appointed Commissioner of the Board of Hurt and Sick Sailors. When used as an object lesson illustrating the failures of insufficiently rapid innovation adoption, the story usually focuses on how Lind's *Treatise on Scurvy*[3] unfortunately failed to convince a troglodyte, penny-pinching Admiralty Board. It was only later, when the more scientifically minded Blane took charge, that the proper policy was implemented.

The Doctor and the Algorithm. S. Scott Graham, Oxford University Press. © Oxford University Press 2022.
DOI: 10.1093/oso/9780197644461.003.0004

As you might expect, the real story is a bit more complicated. Lind's *Treatise on Scurvy* is a massive 456-page tome that reports on the then-current state of scientific knowledge. It addresses all manner of provisional theories, including the possible hereditary causes of scurvy and the potential difference between land- and sea-based varieties of the illness. Along the way, the *Treatise* shares details from a small observational study of 12 shipboard scurvy patients. The 12 patients were divided into six groups of two, and each pair was prescribed a different treatment. Each of five pairs was assigned one of the following: a quart of cider; three doses of elixir vitriol (alcohol and sulfuric acid); three doses of vinegar; an unknown quantity of sea water; and a concoction of nutmeg, garlic, mustard seed, cream of tartar, and myrrh suspended in a mixture of barley water and aromatic tree sap. And, of course, one lucky pair got "two oranges and one lemon."[4] Although, this was top-tier science for the era, it is perhaps understandable that the Admiralty did not immediately overhaul naval policy based on a small observational study buried in a massive tome describing all things scurvy.

A few years later, Lind published a sort of practical guide to naval medicine under the title *An Essay on the Most Effectual Means of Preserving the Health of Seamen, in the Royal Navy.*[5] This more economical 119-page volume was designed as a science-based guide to all manner of illness and injury that might be encountered by a ship's physician. While this primer still did not result in any citrus-based policy changes, it does appear to have been well received by at least some members of the naval medical community. In fact, Blane was so impressed by the volume that in 1780 he prepared a sort of CliffsNotes version under the title *A Short Account of the Most Effectual Means of Preserving the Health of Seamen, Particularly in the Royal Navy.*[6] Blane's more efficient 67-page pamphlet distilled the insights of Lind's scholarly oeuvre and combined those insights with reports of similar experiments by Captain James Cook. While Blane's aggregation of the available evidence usefully advanced the medical science and shipboard clinical practice of the day, as mentioned above it still did not result in policy change. Broad adoption of citrus as a prophylactic for scurvy simply did not happen until it had the regulatory force of approval by the Commissioner of the Board of Hurt and Sick Sailors.

At this point, I've spent a fair amount of time talking about 18th-century medicine for a book on AI. I do so because, despite the limitations of the apocryphal version, the history of scurvy in the Royal Navy provides a nice distillation of what it takes for medical innovation to make it. Promising evidence, on its own, was not enough. Over the course of 40 years and multiple publications, medical science accumulated a body of evidence that eventually achieved regulatory approval. Multiple scientific reports, practical educational materials, and regulatory decisions all fed into the eventual policy change. While this story is often cited as a cautionary tale of innovation delayed, it might be better understood as an ideal case of careful scrutiny. Innovation adoption is almost always decried as "delayed," yet in contemporary medicine it has never been faster. The combined apparatuses of biomedical publishing, continuing medical education, industry-friendly regulators, and high-powered marketing make it such that the successful promulgation of a new medical technology is arguably easier than ever before. (Just imagine how much faster the Royal Navy might have changed policies if Lind were working with Big Citrus.) Indeed, there is a growing body of evidence that the rapid pace of adoption is leading to unprecedented "medical reversal"—where newly adopted clinical practices are actually more harmful than the preexisting standard.[7]

Whether an improved technology or a medical reversal, broad innovation adoption is almost always the goal. Given the hype that surrounds AI, it is no wonder that deep medicine futurists want to see it everywhere. And, indeed, to the extent that it might (at least sometimes) improve patient health, we all should want to see innovative technologies take hold. But, of course, this is not just technological panacea rhetoric run amok. Innovation adoption, at its core, is about market share. As the second-to-last chapter in *Artificial Intelligence in Medicine* puts it, "market adoption defines success."[8] Deep medicine is big business, and there are significant potential revenues on the line. Correspondingly, there are real concerns that these potential revenues may drive hasty adoption and subsequent medical reversal. So, if innovation adoption has gone from maybe too slow to almost certainly too fast, it is critical that we know how new medical technologies are promulgated. In the context of deep medicine, we must better understand the processes by which a new AI becomes portable and makes it. Subsequently, in what follows I explore two cases of innovation promulgation in health AI. The first case focuses on an assistive AI designed to support mammography interpretation, and the second explores a new automated system for diagnosing onychomycosis (toenail fungus). But first, I will take a brief moment to explore the culture of disruptive innovation that drives much of the technology industry. Doing so is a critical first step in understanding how deep medicine may lead to increased medical reversal.

DISRUPTIVE INNOVATION AND HEALTH AI

"Move fast and break things," the now-retired internal motto of Facebook, Inc., exemplifies the culture of disruptive innovation and technochauvinism. The term "disruptive innovation" was coined in a 1995 *Harvard Business Review* article by Joseph Bower and Clayton Christensen.[9] While "innovation," without the modifier "disruptive," might be discussed primarily in terms of novelty, discovery, and even user needs, "disruptive innovation" centers firmly on market share. Fundamentally, disruptive innovation is about shifting established firms out of their dominant market position and generating rapid profit with a new or seemingly new innovation. The dangers of disruptive innovation for technology broadly and AI specifically have received considerable attention in both scholarly and news media circles. In the wake of the Facebook / Cambridge Analytic scandal, for example, many were quick to point out that "Facebook can't move fast enough . . . to fix the things it broke."[10] Indeed, the recent emergence and growing influence of critical algorithm studies is largely a response to the many failures of disruptive innovation. Tech company after tech company moved so fast that they broke things (and people). At the very least, disruptive innovation has been shown frequently to maintain the ongoing breaking of things (and people). Facebook helped to put democracy on a precipice. PredPol has occluded and quite possibly accelerated racism in the prison-industrial complex. Uber built a self-driving car that killed Elaine Herzberg. The adverse effects (both intended and unintended) of AI have been well documented in critical algorithm studies and the popular media. I won't (and quite frankly can't) review it all here. Nevertheless, there are certain cultural similarities between disruptive innovation in tech and disruptive innovation in deep medicine that must be addressed here.

Broussard's *Artificial Unintelligence* traces many of the problems of technochauvinism and tech culture back to its origins in mathematics and computer science. Specifically, she notes that Silicon Valley "inherited mathematicians' worship of the cult genius," which has led to continued "enforce[ment] of the boundaries of industry and camouflage[ing] of structural discrimination."[11] AI (as a tech culture) is, of course, a near seamless overlap between industry and academic computer science. It is quite common to find scholars with university affiliations working at Google and Ph.D.-holding Google employees publishing in top-tier scholarly journals. Across both sectors,

> we have a small, elite group of men who tend to overestimate their mathematical abilities, who have systematically excluded women and people of color in favor of machines for centuries, who tend to want to make science fiction real, who have little regard for social convention, who don't believe that social norms or rules apply to them, who have unused piles of government money sitting around, and who have adopted the ideological rhetoric of far-right libertarian anarcho-capitalists. What could possibly go wrong?[12]

While Broussard's encapsulation of tech and computer science broadly certainly does not describe all of deep medicine, there are plenty of areas of overlap.

Deep medicine is routinely offered up as a form of disruptive innovation that cannot arrive fast enough. Topol, for example, details how AI might help us overcome the many problems of medicine. In so doing, he paints a

dark picture of contemporary American medicine, one dominated by bu-
reaucracy, overworked healthcare providers, and insufficient patient care.
And, indeed, it is hard to argue with his diagnoses. Certainly, there are
many significant challenges facing healthcare today. However, invoking
the logic of innovation adoption, he chastises the medical community for
its failure to embrace the transformative change of AI. As Topol writes,

> We're early in the AI medicine era; it's not routine medical practice
> and some call it "Silicon Valley-dation." Such dismissive attitudes are
> common in medicine, making change in the field glacial. The re-
> sult here is that although most sectors of the world are well into the
> Fourth Industrial Revolution, which is centered on the use of AI,
> medicine is still stuck in the early phase of the third, which is to say,
> the first widespread use of computers.[13]

Here, his criticism parallels the parable of scurvy. Topol casts the early
pioneers of deep medicine as the modern misunderstood James Linds. In
so doing, Topol adopts the mantle of Gilbert Blaine, hoping to catalyze a
more enthusiastic embrace of AI and in so doing disrupt the dominant
practices of medicine.

Representatives from the health tech industry are, of course, happy to
adopt this narrative. Treating medicine as a recalcitrant culture that fails to
adequately recognize the value of new innovations helps to frame AI as a
necessary evolution in medicine science. In the aforementioned "Industry
Perspectives" chapter from *Artificial Intelligence in Medicine*, the authors
lament the many impediments to innovation adoption, "Regulatory, patient safety, workflow, cost, infrastructure, human resources, and others
can all be enormous barriers for a new technology to be implemented
within hospitals."[14] In so doing, they also decry the overall failure of medicine to appreciate innovation: "You will not be surprised to see healthcare seems stuck 15 years or more behind other industries when it comes
to adopting new technologies."[15] Here, we must remember that "success,"
from the industry perspective, is fundamentally about market share. Saved
lives, improved patient outcomes, improved hospital efficiencies, and the

like all take a backseat to the idea that AI success is AI adoption. And, fundamentally, "adoption" means sales:

> After a commercial launch of a new application, adoption became one of the most important parameters to evaluate success. In the start-up and investment world the product—market fit is an essential term, because it has an important feature to predict the potential adoption speed and rate before the official product launch.[16]

Market share is the measure of innovation. The logic of discovery is folded seamlessly into a marketing rhetoric that merges cutting-edge science with an aggressive approach to sales.[17] And, as emerging research on medical reversal shows us, the results can be quite dangerous.

In their aforementioned article on medical reversal, Vinay Prasad and Adam Cifu distinguish between *replacement* and *reversal*.[18] Replacement is what we hope always happens as medical science progresses, namely, that scientific innovation leads to improved patient care. In their later book on the subject, Prasad and Cifu point to obvious historical examples such as where "antibiotics have replaced arsenic, and anesthesia has replaced a bullet held bracingly between the teeth."[19] Reversal (as opposed to re-placement) is where an inferior approach replaces a better preestablished technique. *Ending Medical Reversal* offers a litany of examples, most of which were curated for their audience of healthcare practitioners. Two of the more widely known include the regular mammography screening and the pain killer Vioxx. Despite years of advice to the contrary, routine mammography in women under 50 has limited potential for saving lives and can result in considerable harms ranging from unneeded biopsies to unnecessary prophylactic mastectomies.[20] As a result, a number of major medical organizations no longer recommend annual screening as a matter of course in younger age rages.[21] As it turns out, the previous standard of care was better. Vioxx, once famous for being the exciting new innovation of choice among nonsteroidal anti-inflammatory drugs (NSAIDs), ended up causing severe heart damage in a significant number of patients.[22] Before its recall, Vioxx is estimated to have caused about 140,000 heart attacks and 60,000 deaths.[23] It turns out that many patients would have done just as well taking long-standing and well-established over-the-counter NSAIDs such as ibuprofen or naproxen sodium.

Importantly, unnecessary surgeries and serious adverse events are not required to meet the standards for "medical reversal." Prasad and Cifu take a broad view of harms. They point to the value of comparative clinical effectiveness research that includes costs to patients as critical to investigating medical reversal. In short, if two drugs are equally likely to help patients and have no difference in side effects, cost becomes a critical concern. If one of these two essentially identical drugs costs $12 a dose and the other $250 a dose, the former is the better option. Given this broad understanding of harms, it is critical to note that if a new drug is no better than an old drug but costs more, that still counts as medical reversal. Like many other critics of the contemporary pharmaceutical industry, Prasad and Cifu point to marketing and advertising practices as a key cause for concern. They note that direct-to-consumer (DTC) marketing often "create[s] interest in a new, generally more expensive product . . ."[24]

Likewise, as they note in the original article, "Financial incentives are strongly aligned to promote new technologies."[25] Industry funding of medical research, financial conflicts of interests held by researchers and doctors, and venture capital investments all drive perturbations in medical research that can lead to overly enthusiastic portrayals of technological innovation. The logics of disruptive innovation drive medical technologies to pursue forever the displacement of standard practices with new technologies that may be replacement and may be reversal. This is probably the most dangerous aspect of hype in deep medicine. Certainly, there are many promising technologies that may offer important improvements in patient care and that may lead to appropriate replacement of current standards of care. Once again, separating the promise from the peril becomes a truly fraught (but essential) endeavor. As *The Doctor and the Algorithm* continues to work at this problem, the remainder of this chapter is devoted to better understanding the mechanisms of innovation dissemination in deep medicine. As mentioned above, I do so through exploring twin cases in diagnostic AI—one involving mammography, the other toenail fungus.

Importantly, my focus will be on the practices of innovation dissemination. Along the way, I am mindful of the perils of reversal, but I cannot claim that these are clearly cases of reversal in action. It is very possible that they are replacement. This, too, points to the challenge of separating the promise from the peril in deep medicine. Discriminating between replacement and reversal is often a retrospective judgment. It's much harder to find that line with new innovations on offer in real time.[26]

INTERPENETRATING PORTABILITY ENGINES

As mentioned in Chapter 1, the processes of blackboxing provide the requisite preconditions for portability and (misplaced) trust. By occluding the complex sociotechnical systems that compose an AI, that AI is rendered a thing, a product. It is thus packaged and ready for dissemination, distribution, and prognostication. Of course, as the rhetorics of innovation dissemination and disruptive innovation make clear, many "novel" technologies are not taken up, or at least not taken up quickly. To extend the metaphor of the black box, packaging a product is not enough. The linguistic equivalents of supply chain logistics are required to ensure that the product "moves in space."[27] As described above, the more complete tale of citrus adoption in the Royal Navy provides a convenient illustration of the key engines of portability in health technology: (1) scientific dissemination, (2) (continuing) medical education, (3) marketing, and (4) regulatory approval. For an AI to make it, the blackboxed thing must successfully travel each of these interpenetrating sociotechnical networks. Effective approaches to portability (potentially securing market share) require the careful and integrated management of scientific journal articles, medical symposia and conferences, professional and patient advertising systems, and FDA approval mechanisms.

One might imagine that these different portability engines were arrayed sequentially. That is, in an ideal world, scientific dissemination and scrutiny would precede regulatory approval, which would in turn precede medical education and marketing. Unfortunately, we don't live in that ideal world. Medical science, education, and marketing are often deeply interpenetrated, especially in the advance of disruptive innovation. To be sure, there is a wealth of research available demonstrating the sophistication and reach of marketing for medical innovation. Dominique Tobbell's *Pills, Power, and Policy*, Joseph Gabriel's *Medical Monopoly*, Marcia Angell's *The Truth about Drug Companies*, Carl Elliott's *Better than Well* and his *White Coat, Black Hat* provide countless examples of how biomedical marketing has successfully integrated scientific research, medical education, patient advocacy, regulatory decision-making, and legislative practices. In some cases, at least, it is no different in health AI. In what follows, I explore the integrated marketing and communication (marcom) strategy of one health technology firm that has developed a radiology decision support AI for breast cancer detection.[28]

iCAD Inc is a health technology company based in San Jose, California. Their signature product is ProFound AI™. The application suite provides a range of AI-driven diagnostic and decision support tools primarily built around imaging technologies for breast cancer detection, e.g., mammography and tomosynthesis. ProFound AI™ is noteworthy for being one of the first diagnostic AI systems to secure FDA clearance.[29] iCAD describes their product as follows:

> ProFound AI ™ for 2D Mammography and Tomosynthesis. Precise, Powerful & Proven Technology iCAD, the market leader in multivendor computer-aided detection of breast cancer with more than 4,000 installations worldwide, introduces the latest in artificial intelligence—ProFound AI. ProFound AI is a precise, powerful and proven deep learning, artificial intelligence platform that assists radiologists with reading 2D mammography and breast tomosynthesis.[30]

Here, in an overtly promotional context, we find the standard appeals to precision mixed with more typical marketing claims about broad innovation adoption "4,000 installations worldwide" and innovation "the latest in artificial intelligence." Of course, iCAD's marketing is not just about buzzwords. AI marketing is grounded in essentially the same appeals to measured precision that we find in the scientific literature.

However, before we dive into the rhetoric of iCAD's PR, it is important to get an overall lay of the land. As mentioned earlier, pharmaceutical and health technology companies have become experts in integrated marketing communication (marcom) initiatives that advance their technologies and maximize sales. U.S. federal law (and counterparts in the EU and other national governments) requires a scientific foundation for healthcare technology. This means that potential buyers and users (doctors, hospitals, etc.) are trained to look for certain forms of evidence in certain types of venues in order to evaluate the quality of new technologies. Health technology companies and the specialty PR firms they hire are keenly aware of this. Thus, success in making AI (or any other healthcare product really) is about deploying an integrated scientific-marcom strategy. Figure 3.1 is an illustrative model of iCAD's approach for ProFound AI™. As we can see, there are three major tracks in iCAD's strategy: a regulatory track, a scientific track, and a sales track. While one might imagine that these tracks function independently, they are highly integrated in practice.

Following federal regulations, scientific inquiry is the basic foundation of iCAD's marcom strategy. The results of that scientific inquiry were first submitted to the FDA by way of what's called a 510(k) application. 510(k) is a sort of expedited application process whereby new medical devices can

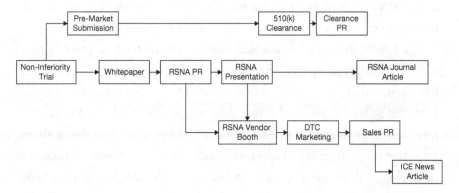

Figure 3.1. An illustration of iCAD's integrated marcom strategy. RSNA = Radiological Society of North America; ICE = Imaging Conference & Expo.

be cleared for market if they can demonstrate substantial equivalence to an existing technology.[31] 510(k) regulatory clearance is a lower bar than "approval" but essentially grants the same privileges. Medical devices that present a greater risk to patients (Class III devices) require a higher standard of evaluation and have to be granted "approval" rather than clearance. Pursuant to 510(k) regulations, iCAD's ProFound AI™ benchmarking data is packaged in the form of a non-inferiority trial.[32] Non-inferiority trials are designed to evaluate whether a new product or practice is "not worse" than an existing product or practice. Non-inferiority trials are frequently contrasted with the more familiar "superiority trials," which aim to demonstrate that a product is superior to a placebo. Interestingly, iCAD's trial design actually assesses the non-inferiority of a radiologist using ProFound AI™ compared with a radiologist not using ProFound AI™. In so doing, iCAD embodies what both proponents and detractors alike recommend as the best possible version of AI—the so-called Third Wave AI. Third Wave AI does not replace humans so much as it assists them. It augments human expertise by drawing on a broader range of experiences than any given human can bring to bear. Yet, the human is still ultimately in charge of the decision-making. Even strident AI critic Broussard is quick to note that "humans plus machines outperforms humans alone or machines alone."[33] Topol, too, recommends a Third Wave approach for deep medicine. He envisions a world where "doctors will adopt AI and algorithms as their work partners."[34] Importantly, most current FDA-approved health AI devices are Third Wave and generally require "clinicians to confirm information provided . . . and to be responsible for decisions."[35]

Since 1985, the FDA has allowed non-inferiority trials in place of more traditional superiority trials for drug and device approval,[36] a policy that has been widely criticized. Notably, non-inferiority trials have a strong potential to lead to medical reversal. Even the most well-conducted non-inferiority trials are likely to lead to marketing a product that, despite being no better (non-inferior), is more expensive than the current standard. In reference to drug development in oncology, Prasad argues that "non-inferiority trials should only be run for drugs that are either (1) cheaper, (2) more convenient, or (3) less toxic than older ones."[37] Unfortunately, current usage of non-inferiority trial designs is rather more expansive. Despite these criticisms, non-inferiority trials are essentially the required approach for 510(k) approval.

Shortly after pre-marketing submission, but before clearance, iCAD began its public-facing integrated marcom strategy. Without FDA clearance or approval, it is illegal to actually market a new device, and so traditional advertising materials do not start to emerge until shortly after approval. However, pre-clearance scientific reporting is certainly allowed. Thus, iCAD's marcom efforts began with an abbreviated white paper reporting trial results[38] and an academic presentation delivered at the 2018 Radiological Society of North America (RSNA) annual meeting. The presentation was delivered by the study's lead researcher, Emily Conant, Professor of Radiology at the Hospital of the University of Pennsylvania. Shortly before the presentation, iCAD issued a press release announcing the upcoming talk and highlighting the location of their vendor booths at RSNA.[39]

510(k) clearance[40] and a related press release[41] followed not long after the RSNA presentation. DTC marketing arrived fast on the heels of clearance with targeted websites[42] and brochures.[43] As mentioned earlier, the non-inferiority trial and related benchmarking were the cornerstone of iCAD's promotional efforts. While it is possible to locate the radiologist with and radiologist without accuracy metrics, the data highlighted most clearly in marketing materials is the comparative improvement for radiologists using ProFound AI™. The product brochure, for example, highlights both clinical performance and workflow benefits, both of which were assessed in the trial. Specifically, the various scientific and marketing products highlight an 8.0% increase in sensitivity, a 6.9% increase in specificity, and a 5.7% improvement in AUC scores. Under workflow benefits, iCAD focuses on data indicating that using ProFound AI™ can result in a 52.7% reduction in the amount of time radiologists spend reading diagnostic images.

Reduced time-on-task for expensive radiologists is a key feature of iCAD's marketing strategy. In the published white paper, reading time is offered as one of two co-primary research objectives alongside non-inferiority. While the modest increases in accuracy might be a boon to patient health, there's no doubt that such a significant reduction in reading time can translate into big money for hospitals. Theoretically, a radiologist focusing on mammography and tomosynthesis could double her daily caseload with ProFound AI™. Much in the way of critical algorithm studies, this kind of profit maximization was found to be a central feature of AI marketing and hype. As Benjamin notes,

> Computational approaches to a wide array of problems are seen as not only good but necessary, and make feature of cost-cutting measures in the outsourcing of decisions to "smart" machines. Whether deciding which teacher to hire or fire or which loan applicant to approve or decline, automated systems are alluring because they seem to remove the burden from gatekeepers, who may be too overworked or too biased to make sound judgments.[44]

Freeing up healthcare providers from the mundane while maximizing profits was also a key affordance offered by Topol. Reducing time-on-task and potentially cost of care could be great in a U.S. context, but only if the products work as well as expected and promote patient health across communities. Unfortunately, that "across communities" part is a real deficit in much of AI, and ProFound AI™ appears to be no exception.

Interestingly, it would be almost nine months after 510(k) clearance before a full report on the non-inferiority trial would be published in RSNA's journal, *Radiology-Artificial Intelligence*.[45] The 2018 white paper, which had previously been the most comprehensive source of data on the study, focused primarily on endpoints and outcomes. It left out critical information about study design that is usually considered essential to scientific reporting. Even more importantly, no data presentation I could find provides any information about participant demographics. In a larger study of similar techniques published a few months earlier in *JAMA-Oncology*, Conant and her coauthors provided demographic data and noted that "data came from health care systems in the northeastern United States. Minority and Hispanic women were underrepresented, and most women had health insurance."[46] It is interesting and unfortunate that research in two related studies led by the same scientist—the one directly supporting a marketed device—fails to include demographic data or even acknowledge the potential limitations of a potentially inappropriately diverse training set.[47]

As Figure 3.1 details, another important aspect of iCAD's marcom strategy is vendor booths at national meetings. The RSNA is one of the signature radiology meetings in North America. Like all such meetings, it is a mix of scholarly presentations, research posters, continuing education, and vendor fairs. Radiology researchers, practitioners, and professionals attend RSNA to find out about the latest advances, but also to maintain their licensure through continuing education. In technology-heavy fields like radiology, the vendor fair is an important way for practitioners and administrators to learn about the latest products. It is also big business. Before it was canceled for COVID, RSNA 2020 was charging $6,500 for a basic kiosk and $12,500 for a deluxe kiosk in the AI Showcase.[48] It is not uncommon for several hundred vendors to hawk their wares at such conferences. Another meeting where iCAD takes out vendor space is the annual meeting of The Imaging Conference & Expo or ICE, as they call themselves despite being unrelated to a certain federal law enforcement agency.[49] At face value, ICE and the ICE community look like the RSNA. It is an annual conference for radiologists, radiology technicians, and hospital administrators. It offers continuing medical education certified by the American Society of Radiologic Technologists (ASRT) and, in some years, Accreditation Council in Imaging (ACI, the accreditation body of the European Board of Radiology). As it turns out, ICE is a subsidiary of MD Publishing, Inc., a trade press and specialty PR firm that serves the medical device industry. Catalogs, trade expos, and industry magazines appear to be the bread and butter of MD Publishing, Inc. I mention ICE and MD Publishing, Inc., because I noted that they are quick to pick up on industry press releases. In fact, they recently ran an article[50] on impressive iCAD sales following a release on that topic.[51]

While I certainly have no evidence to indicate that ProFound AI is a case of medical reversal, a tour of iCAD's integrated marcom strategy shows the many vectors whereby the integrity of innovation and dissemination

processes might be influenced by financial interests. The scientific reporting and medical education are timed perfectly to correspond to regulatory approval, and the end result is that innovation dissemination and
adoption are essentially contemporaneous. iCAD has solved the scurvy
problem by compressing the networks of scientific security, regulatory approval, and medical education into a singularity. The approach appears to
have the desired effects in terms of market share—four thousand licenses
and counting according to the most recent marketing materials. Once
again, I stress that it is certainly possible that iCAD's technology offers a
case study in replacement rather than reversal. We may well see improved
patient outcomes following this broad adoption. However, the rapidity
of the progress from initial dissemination to broad usage makes the saga
of James Lind, perhaps, a bit more appealing. Indeed, Lind's initial study
noted that a quart of cider was nearly as efficacious as citrus fruit. Without
Cook's confirmatory findings, a rush to judgment at the Board of Hurt and
Sick Sailors may have resulted in the Royal Navy adopting this cheaper
and ineffective remedy. Regardless of the particulars of Lind or iCAD, it
is increasingly troubling that speed of adoption is so often presented as an
unqualified good in health technology.

AN OPEN SCIENCE ALTERNATIVE

"Open science" means many things to many different people. Ultimately,
it is a constellation of ethical commitments related to ensuring that scientific research, data, and findings are available to all. The most recent
iterations of open science have emerged out of the open access movement, an approach to democratizing knowledge that centers on dropping
economic barriers (chiefly paywalls) to scientific reporting. The famous
FOSTER taxonomy identifies four primary movements that comprise
open science: open access, open data, open source, and open reproducible
research.[52] Later efforts in open science add open notebooks, open peer review, open network, open educational resources, and citizen science to the
broad umbrella of open science.[53] Importantly, open science is not new,

nor is it new to medical science. Jonas Salk famously refusing to patent the polio vaccine is a classic example of open science. In fact, the American pharmaceuticals industry was largely devoted to open science from its inception until the early 1900s. Joseph Gabriel's *Medical Monopoly* offers a detailed tour of the long history of self-described "ethical" pharmacists who were committed to open formulary and anti-monopolistic trade practices.[54] Open science (like open access or open source) is largely about disrupting monopolistic practices that inhibit the free flow of information. Open science is about disrupting the very idea of market position by ensuring that all may benefit from the insights of scientific research. Open science is supported by open access journals (that never charge a subscription fee), online data repositories that make the stuff of scientific inquiry accessible and downloadable, and coding repositories like GitHub that allow anyone with the requisite knowledge to use, modify, and improve open-source software.

Ultimately, the open science movement provides an interesting counterexample to typical narratives of industry-driven innovation dissemination. To be sure, blackboxing and portability remain central concerns to making an AI and an AI that makes it. Thus, you will see much of the same communication and even marketing activity associated with more traditional industry technologies. However, open science walks an interesting line between blackboxing a technology and leaving it open to scrutiny. A novel AI system must be blackboxed and thingified if it is to be portable, but a fully open science product is never entirely closed. The pinnacle of black boxed technology are those devices that come with heavy-handed warnings about voiding your warranty if you open the black box. The black boxes of open science might be a little bit more like birthday presents. To be sure, they are boxed and wrapped, but they come with an invitation to see what is inside.

By way of illustration, I turn to a 2018 *PLOS One* article entitled "Deep Neural Networks Show an Equivalent and Often Superior Performance to Dermatologists in Onychomycosis Diagnosis: Automatic Construction of Onychomycosis Datasets by Region-Based Convolutional Deep Neural Network."[55] In this study, the authors use a reginal convoluted neural network (R-CNN) to develop an automated onychomycosis (toenail fungus) diagnostic system. They offer this system not as a total replacement for specialty dermatology, but rather as a useful addition to the "telemedicine environment where the access to dermatologists is unavailable."[56] This is another example of Third Wave AI. In this case the goal is to provide something more akin to specialty dermatology knowledge in a more general clinical environment. An interesting addition to their development process in this context is that the system is shown to be rather accurate even with poor-quality smartphone photos such as those that might be taken by patients themselves. In an environment where access to care is inequitably distributed (e.g., the United States), this could indeed be an asset.

The developed R-CNN system works in two successive stages, first identifying finger and toenails and then looking for signs of disease. The two-stage process is essential because clinical imagines include a lot of things that might be toenails but are not toenails. Identifying toes as toes and toenails as toenails is a critical prerequisite for discriminating between what might be healthy, decorated, or smashed—none of which is onychomycosis.[57] The successful subsampling and feature mapping of the R-CNN is what makes diagnostics possible. Nails are filtered from bodies and contexts and then parsed for features that may indicate fungus-driven disease processes. One of the benefits of R-CNN systems (as opposed to the SVM architecture discussed in Chapter 1) is that they do not require targeted feature engineering prior to modeling. However, this comes with its own downside. When computers learn by example, they often need many examples. As the authors note, "CNN systems become more accurate as the data volumes get larger."[58] Thus, this nail fungus diagnostic system was developed with an initial data set of 598,854 clinical images. The development team was able to use a preexisting R-CNN-based hand-and-foot image selector to extract 42,981 pictures of hands and feet from the larger data set. Then a dermatologist hand-annotated a subsample of 3,741 images to identify finger- and toenails. Finally, a team of three dermatologists labeled nail images with one of six classes: onychomycosis, nail dystrophy, onycholysis, melanonychia, normal, and other.[59] The authors fed these data into two different R-CNN architectures, VGG-19 and ResNet-152. The details are beyond the scope of this chapter, but those numbers at the end indicate the number of layers in each CNN, 19 and 152, respectively. The outputs of the VGG-19 and ResNet-152 networks were ensembled (combined) into a single output with a binary diagnosis (onychomycosis or not).[60] The authors evaluated their approach using several different data sets. Throughout the results section of the article, they report sensitivity, specificity, AUC, and the Youden index scores. Again, the more fine-grained details of these metrics are not critical to the current chapter. However, the overall investment in benchmarking is. Reporting accuracy results takes up 4 whole pages in a 14-page article.

Over the course of the article, the disaggregated pile of 500,000+ images, dermatologists, patient records, and CNN architectures becomes *a* system. Here, the article rehearses the logic of blackboxing discussed in Chapter 1. By detailing the study mechanisms and measurements, the article itself (as an act of scientific communication) reinforces the processes of assessing the system. Also, just as we saw in Chapter 1, once its performativity is established, the complex system that created it is erased. Unsuccessful processes remain open to interrogation. When an AI system doesn't work or isn't understood to work, the processes are put on full display to see if it is possible to make it work. Success, or at least stipulative success, is the primary mechanism whereby sociotechnical systems are blackboxed. This is precisely the affordance provided by the many metrics of ML.

The portability of black boxes is evident in how they are taken up in future research. The conventions of scholarly writing, including citation practices, provide a ready-made framework for accepting the blackboxing produced by the original article. A few examples from the citation history of Han et al.'s article are sufficient to make the point. A 2020 *Skin Research and Technology* article declares that "Han established a convolutional neural network model for recognizing onychomycosis, and the accuracy rate reached that of dermatologists" (p. 5).[61] In so doing, the article accepts the black box as ready-made. In fact, this example is noteworthy in that it recognizes the agency of Han's team at all. "Established" implies a process, albeit a process that is complete. A 2018 study from *Progress in Retinal and Eye Research* grants all agency to the technology itself: "In another dermatological application, onychomycosis diagnosis, a CNN performed equally to or better than a panel of dermatologists with various skill levels doing the same assessment in a painstaking manual fashion (Han et al., 2018)" (p. 4).[62] A significant indicator of successful blackboxing is to be nominalized in batch citation. A 2020 *British Journal of Dermatology* article does just this when it notes that "DCNNs that can classify dermatological diseases at a standard equivalent to a board-certified dermatologist have been reported.[12-17]" (p. 182).[63] As citation #13, Han et al. aren't even visible on the page, yet here the acceptance of their success is unambiguous all the same.

This tour of subsequent citations shows us how blackboxing was a successful guarantor of portability. Yet, at the same time, as an act of open science, Han et al.'s article resists closure. Ultimately, the study embodies many of the core commitments of open science. It is published in an open access journal sponsored by the Public Library of Science, a leader in the open access movement. Additionally, the authors have made their validation training sets, CNN models, and code freely available to all. In short, you can pick your way through every last bit of the assemblage, unboxing as you go. This especially impressive commitment to transparency also provides the necessary foundation to reinvent their R-CNN, an important opportunity given one of the key flaws of the study—the limited diversity of the training data.

Unlike the WBCD discussed in Chapter 1, the data used to development the toenail fungus R-CNN system are not entirely without demographics. However, only age and gender statistics are provided. Training data were collected from several major South Korean hospitals. The Korean population is 96% ethnically Korean. Therefore, it is probably safe to assume that data collected from clinical records at Korean hospitals are mostly from ethnically Korean patients. While I have not surveyed the full data set, it is noteworthy that none of the sample images provided in the article appear to show Black or brown skin. As Benjamin reminds us, "To the extent that machine learning relies on large, 'naturally occurring' datasets that are rife with racial (and economic and gendered) biases, the raw data that robots are using to learn and make decisions about the world reflect deeply ingrained cultural prejudices and structural hierarchies."[64] Of course, AI is not the only context in which these biases operate. Dermatology—writ large—is in the early stages of a reckoning on this issue as increasing bodies of research demonstrate that dermatological images are overwhelming white or light-skinned.[65] Insofar as the basic software and code have been provided to any users, it would be entirely possible to replicate this study on a more diverse data set or on a data set that is more representative of communities served by a given clinic or hospital system. Importantly, using this software does not require an ongoing subscription, as is the case with ProFoundAI™.

MAKING AN AI THAT MAKES IT

Combining the insights from the three case studies from this chapter and Chapter 1, we can work our way to a general map of the sociotechnical systems that support blackboxing and black box portability. Figure 3.2

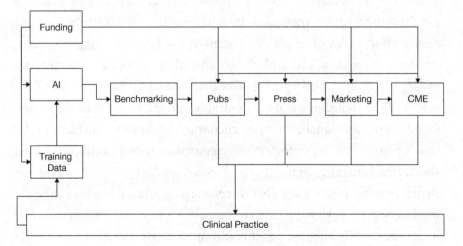

Figure 3.2. The Sociotechnical network for making AI.

illustrates this network. There are multiple pathways articulated in this network, and not all will be activated in any given cases. The iCAD promotional network makes use of all the connects. The open science network of the toenail fungus R-CNN uses fewer. Nevertheless, two key issues are central. The overall shape of the network is circular. Health AI development draws from current clinical practice to create standardized data sets against which benchmarking can occur. In some cases, like the WBCD, the data are canonical. In other cases, researchers curate their own data sets like the toe fungus data images that drive Han et al.'s R-CNN system or the radiologist readings of mammograms and tomosynthesis imaging that were used to train ProFound AI™. The processes of AI development and blackboxing serve to concretize the decisions made in these curated data sets and relay them with speed and scale back onto future clinical practice. This essentially circular dynamic is a double-edged sword. If training data is well-selected and well-curated, then it can support substantially improved clinical practice. However, the circularity of the system is precisely why so much in AI serves to concretize and accelerate inequitable structures. Implicit biases in the training data are established as "The Reference" against which good clinical practice should be measured.

The other critical item to notice here is the centrality of benchmarking. Benchmarking is essentially what old-school actor–network theorists would call an "obligatory passage point." Making an AI that makes it requires successfully traversing this particular node. Whether an industry effort or an open science initiative, the benchmarking process is critical to what makes AI a black box and what authorizes it to circulate in larger sociotechnical systems. Good scores with quality metrics support 510(k) applications and are central to integrated marcom strategies. Good scores with quality metrics encourage healthcare providers to dig into open-source repositories and repurpose useful technologies. In short, benchmarking makes both blackboxing and portability possible. Benchmarking metrics are also of central importance because they are used to assess the extent to which one practice is superior (or non-inferior) to another. Well-designed benchmarking methods should vouchsafe for a new product and stand in the way of medical reversal. Subsequently, benchmarking warrants further serious scrutiny. And this is the task of Chapter 4. In the next chapter, I will offer a deep dive into accuracy and validity metrics used in AI development. In so doing, I explore some of the underdiscussed limitations of these metrics and their common deployment in health AI.

The Search for Ground Truth

In 2012, 52-year-old Tasleem Rafiq suddenly collapsed in her home in Reading, United Kingdom. Her family was with her at the time and immediately called emergency services. An ambulance was dispatched, and on arrival paramedics began emergency resuscitation. Rafiq had suffered a heart attack and was transported to Royal Berkshire Hospital where resuscitation efforts continued. After 45 minutes without success, she was pronounced dead. Eleven hours later, Tasleem Rafiq woke up.[1] At the time, doctors were sure that her ordeal would result in irrevocable brain injury. Nevertheless, Rafiq made what is often described as a "miraculous recovery" and has since returned to her normal life. Rafiq's story is rare but not unique. Every few years, the media will report another case of miraculous recovery. In 2020, Timesha Beauchamp, of Michigan, made it all the way to the funeral home before she was found, still breathing, in a body bag.[2] Unfortunately, her story doesn't have a happy ending. Beauchamp eventually died due to the lack of care she received.

Although these stories make the news with some regularity, cases of autoresuscitation or "Lazarus syndrome" are extremely uncommon. A 2007 review of the literature found a total of 38 documented cases.[3] Nevertheless, I draw attention to these cases because they do, in fact, exist. While "autoresuscitation" describes the physiological mechanisms involved, what we are actually looking at here are cases of misdiagnosed death. It hardly seems like such a thing should be possible. Death should be the most obvious and clear of diagnoses. In 1789, Benjamin Franklin

The Doctor and the Algorithm. S. Scott Graham, Oxford University Press. © Oxford University Press 2022.
DOI: 10.1093/oso/9780197644461.003.0005

famously described it as one of only two certain things in this world—the other being taxes. However, the simple truth of the matter is that no decision-making process is 100% accurate. Medicine is simply not infallible.

This is not news, of course. No one who has ever paid any attention to medicine at all might imagine that it could be infallible. However, we are often quick to ascribe fallibility to aberration. Medicine is thought to be wrong when fallible people make mistakes or succumb to bias. But medicine is fallible even in the best of cases. Our most respected technological conceits fail to achieve 100% accuracy. Let's take an everyday example that most of us are familiar with—the rapid antigen strep test. Strep throat is a relatively common ailment, and a moderate cause for concern, especially in pediatric medicine. As the name suggests, strep throat is a streptococcus (bacterial) infection of the throat and tonsils. Generally, when a healthy immune system is exposed to harmful bacteria or virus, it will produce antigens. Targeted antigens are custom-engineered molecules that are designed to bind to specific bacteria to prevent those bacteria from infecting cells. Since antigens are often targeted, we can use rapid antigen tests to infer the presence of certain bacteria in a patient. There are several rapid antigen tests available for a whole host of bacteria and viruses from strep to SARS-COV-2. Typical rapid antigen tests for strep throat correctly detect people with the disease 86% of the time, and they correctly identify people without the disease 95% of the time.[4] This is an everyday test, used widely in clinical care. It is the foundation for daily decisions in pediatrics and family medicine. It is industry standard, and it has a sensitivity (correct when positive) of 86% and a specificity (correct when negative) of 95%. A crude estimate for the sensitivity of death diagnostics would be 99.99999696% (based on 38 misdiagnoses over a 25-year period at 50 million deaths per year). I can't calculate the specificity without knowing how many people were falsely diagnosed as alive during that same time frame.

So, what's the point of all this? It's not to shatter your faith in modern medicine: 99.99999696% is a hell of a success rate for any decision-making process; 86% sensitivity / 95% specificity is also remarkably accurate. Few diagnostic or predictive processes outside of those governed by a priori probabilities (e.g., coin flips) or Newtonian mechanics are more accurate than medicine. Medicine is a complex sociotechnical system, and humans are complex biocultural creatures. The fact that medicine has achieved these levels of accuracy is actually quite remarkable given the inherent complexities and uncertainties. That said, accuracy in medicine is a pivotal issue for deep medicine. As the previous chapters have discussed, accuracy and the metrics that measure accuracy are central to the processes of making an AI—in both senses of the term. AI systems are blackboxed and established as durable things when they reach certain accuracy benchmarks, and these benchmarks are also the foundations of trust, both appropriate and misplaced. However, the centrality of accuracy and its guarantors requires more detailed engagement with the processes of assessing (and also engineering) accuracy.

"Groundtruthing" is a term of art for the research practices involved in cultivating a data set against which a prototype AI will be measured. To the extent that an AI system has an "architecture," groundtruthing creates the foundation. In supervised machine learning, this often involves using human researchers or clinicians to assign diagnostic labels to cases in a training data set. As the death and strep examples indicate, however, these processes have their own accuracy limitations. What's more, the design of a given groundtruthing exercise (single rater, consensus-based, hierarchical rating teams) can have a significant impact on the quality of the underlying data, the reliability of so-called ground truth, and the foundation for a new AI system. Once "ground truth" is established, AI systems are measured against that "truth" using different metrics optimized for different purposes. Metric choice can have a noticeable impact on how useful a new AI system is seen to be. Finally, insofar as AI systems are benchmarked against less-than-100%-accurate groundtruthing exercises, the reported accuracy of the system elides the limited accuracy of the ground truth. The AI's accuracy metric is based on a presupposition of truth, one frequently known to be false, or at the very least limited, but seldom described as such. Thus, in what follows, I offer a deeper exploration of (1) common approaches to groundtruthing in deep medicine, (2) typical accuracy and reliability metrics in health AI, and (3) an underrecognized problem of "bearing capacity" where the ground truth foundations do not adequately support AI system architecture. Along the way, I point to what all this means for the promise and peril of deep medicine.

GROUNDTRUTHING

Groundtruthing exercises in health AI take many forms. As mentioned in the Introduction, ground truth is never simply found truth. It is always created through some combination of data wrangling and investigational processes; hence, "groundtruthing" is a verb. In this chapter, I will discuss three broad categories of groudtruthing: dredged, engineered, and forged. *Dredged* ground truth is my term for the use of preexisting data. Dredged ground truth in precision medicine usually comes from patent medical records or charts. That is, decisions made through everyday clinical practice are taken to be true. Whatever data exists in the patient's chart will be treated as ground truth for the purposes of AI development. *Engineered* ground truth involves creating labeling data using previously established methods. Labels created from recognized lab tests, validated psychological inventories, and autopsy findings are examples of engineered ground truth. Engineered ground truth is distinct from dredged ground truth in that the data did not exist previously in any sort of database or batch of charts. Finally, *forged* ground truth is my way of referring to AI development where researchers create novel groundtruthing processes. Typically, this involves assembling teams of researchers to read and interpret clinical data. As mentioned above, the truthiness of forged truth is warranted through the same kinds of benchmarking exercises as AI development. The differences between engineered and forged ground truth are more a matter of degree than kind. And, importantly, all modes of groundtruthing are, to a certain extent, stipulative. That is, data, whether dredged, engineered, or forged, are taken to be true.

In 2017, researchers at the Stanford University Medical School developed an AI system that somewhat reliably predicts when patients will die.[5] The AI uses a deep neural network (DNN) framework to mine data from electronic health records (EHRs) and synthesizes that data to pre-dict the date of a patient's death, assuming that date will occur in a 3- to 12-month window following hospital evaluation. The DNN has an aston-ishing accuracy of 93%. This is the perfect exemplar of dredged ground truth. The date of death in patient EHRs is used to train the DNN. These data are dredged up out of the EHRs and submitted to the DNN alongside extracted features (e.g., history of cancer, trauma, heart disease; number of outpatient and inpatient encounters; number of diagnostic scans and tests; etc.). As dredged truth, there's no guarantee of accuracy beyond trust in the processes established by the clinical or hospital system. In this case, it is largely a question of how much you trust the policies and data entry practices at Stanford Hospital or the Lucile Packard Children's Hospital. The 3- to 12-month time horizon makes it substantially less likely that col-lected EHRs will include a misdiagnosed death. Ultimately, given the pre-viously mentioned back-of-the-napkin calculations for the sensitivity of death diagnostics, we can infer that this is a very reliable ground truth.

A typical example of engineered ground truth comes from a 2012 Goethe University study published in *Plos-One*.[6] "Using Support Vector Machines [SVM] with Multiple Indices of Diffusion for Automated Classification of Mild Cognitive Impairment," as the title suggests, describes efforts to develop a SVM system that could automatically identify mild cognitive impairment (MCI) from magnetic resonance imaging (MRI) of the brain. The AI development process is not appreciably different from the methods described in the last chapter. The SVM separates MRI voxel (essentially 3D pixels) data by drawing the most efficient hyperplane. As mentioned above, the groundtruthing process is a perfect exemplar of engineered ground truth. For this study, training data labels (MCI diagnoses) were established by having participants take a canonical psychological inven-tory for MCI—the Mini Mental State Examination (MMSE). The MMSE is quite similar to the Montreal Cognitive Assessment, which became fa-mous in recent years after having been administered to Donald Trump. As you may recall, Trump repeatedly bragged about his intelligence because he could remember the words "Person. Woman. Man. Camera. TV."[7] The MMSE has essentially the same question with the suggested terms "Apple,

Table, Penny."[8] The full details are unimportant to this chapter. It is sufficient to know that MMSE is a widely used and validated diagnostic instrument with a sensitivity of 79.8% and a specificity of 81.3%.[9] Incidentally, these values don't come from the MCI SVM study. Recognized and validated diagnostic instruments are blackboxed much like the validated AIs discussed in Chapter 1. As such, using EHR data or MMSE scores does not usually require or involve reporting any assessments of ground truth accuracy or reliability.

Simply put, forging ground truth involves creating a custom-labeled data set, expressly for the purposes of AI development. When commonly accepted and validated diagnostic instruments are unavailable or impractical, researchers must find ways of assigning their own labels to training data. The methods for doing so are quite various. In the most simplistic of cases, a single rater (usually an expert in the relevant clinical area) will make diagnoses for each instance in the training data. In these cases, the AI systems developed essentially learn to diagnose like that one specific doctor. It is an open question as to whether that individual's expertise and training can be reasonably taken to stand in for all similar doctors. Frequently, it has to do with the complexity of the decision. In Chapter 3, I discussed the development of a nail fungus diagnostic DNN. In this case, a single rater was used to train the part of the algorithm that identifies toenails and fingernails. This is perfectly reasonable. It is appropriate to expect that any given doctor can identify fingers and toes as accurately as any other doctor. When it came to actually diagnosing onychomycosis, the research team appropriately moved to a multi-rater design.

Of course, the number of raters involved is not the only variable in forged ground truth. When more than one doctor or researcher is involved in labeling data, disagreements are nearly inevitable. This is the logic behind getting a second opinion. Diagnostic decisions are complex and uncertain. Uniform agreement is largely not possible, in the absence of other factors. Groundtruthing methodologists have adopted a number of strategies to address disagreement. A simple majority vote is a common technique. Some projects use tie-breaking methods. For example, one team working to develop a new AI that can diagnose cataracts used the following process: "Each image was independently described and labelled by two experienced ophthalmologists, and a third ophthalmologist was consulted in the case of disagreement."[10] Another group of ophthalmologists working on glaucoma diagnostics used a more elaborate tie-breaking protocol:

> Special care was taken in order to create a reference gold standard data set. All the images had a double complete glaucoma evaluation performed by six expert (senior) ophthalmologists and nine non-expert (younger) ophthalmologists using a tele-screening tool. The ophthalmologists with more than five years of experience were considered as experts in this work. In case of disagreement between the two evaluations performed, two glaucoma experts decided the final classification of the image by consensus.[11]

As it turns out, expert "consensus" is a widely invoked technique for groundtruthing and for medical decision-making broadly. However, while consensus engineered ground truth is a widely accepted approach, it is not the panacea it might seem to be.

Put simply, consensus requires the invocation of additional social processes to create unanimity. Diagnosticians do not generally achieve unanimity either as a result of standardized training or even by accident. Typically, consensus forging requires the invocation of deliberative and argumentative processes. A Google AI research team described their consensus engineering as follows: "The reference standard was generated by 3 fellowship-trained retina specialists who first graded images independently and then participated in multiple rounds of adjudication until full consensus was reached."[12] This is fancy language for "we fought about it until we agreed." Now, obviously open debate is essentially the primary method by which science functions, so this might well be an effective strategy in some cases. However, AI research frequently occurs on hierarchical teams. It is not uncommon for supervising physicians, residents, and medical students to work simultaneously on forging ground truth. In these cases, it is quite possible that the power dynamics of the laboratory create the equivalent of a single-rater design (based on the diagnostic opinions of the supervisory physician). Finally, there is one other potential significant problem with unanimity—it should never be trusted in the case of large teams. Statistical analyses of the paradox of unanimity shows that when the number of raters exceeds five, unanimity is almost certainly the result of a compromised process.[13] Occasionally, medical researchers will justify their engineered ground truth on the basis of high unanimity. One lung cancer team boasts that "Images derived from different centers were graded by up to eight radiologists."[14] In this study, it is not entirely clear if unanimity was achieved for all eight radiologists. However, if it was that would be a serious cause for concern.

In a follow-up interview, the senior author on the paper that demonstrated the paradox of unanimity suggested that

> A take-home message of our analysis is that the dissenting voice should be welcomed. A wise committee should accept that difference of opinion and simply record there was a disagreement. The recording of the disagreement is not a negative, but a positive that demonstrates that a systemic bias is less likely.[15]

And this is precisely what happens in the best exemplars of forged groundtruthing. A typical example can be found in a 2018 University Hospital of Zurich study that used a DNN to identify breast cancer in ultrasound images.[16] In this study, ground truth was engineered by showing 192 breast ultrasound images to two of three raters. Each rater would view the image, classify it as benign or malignant, and assign a quantitized malignancy score (1–5). Each of the three raters had different levels of experience. Rater 1 was a resident in diagnostic radiology; Rater 2 was a clinician with three years of experience in breast imaging; and Rater 3 was a fourth-year medical student. Rather than use a tie-breaking or consensus metric, the research team used codified statistical measures of agreement (or reliability) to assess the quality of the labeling process. In this case, inter-rater agreement was evaluated using Lin's concordance correlation coefficient

(CCC), and the results were as follows: R1:R2: CCC = .57; R1:R3: CCC = .46.; R2:R3: CCC = .35. I describe the calculation of these metrics more in the next section. For now, you can think of them as "fair to middling." If a tie-breaking or censuses method had been used, we might assume that the groundtruthing process was highly rigorous. Fortunately, reliability metrics allows us to assess more accurately the quality of labeling practices. Yet, this still is not without its problems. The use of reliability metrics to guarantee forged ground truth is essentially the same practice as the use of accuracy statistics to guarantee AI precision. An important question remains about how groundtruthing reliability relates to AI accuracy. This is the bearing capacity issue I tackle later in this chapter.

A MORASS OF METRICS

So much of deep medicine is guaranteed by metrics designed to vouch for the quality of both groundtruthing and AI predictive processes. Over the last few chapters, I've talked about accuracy, sensitivity, specificity, area under (AU) the receiver operating characteristic (ROC) curve (AUROC or AUC), agreement, concordance, etc. It is past time to offer a more careful explanation of at least a few of the key metrics involved, and that's going to involve some math (sorry!). But, before I get into that math, however, I want to outline the general shape of the argument. Essentially, the next few pages are the CliffsNotes for this section. If math isn't your thing, you can skip from where I talk about Figure 4.1 to the beginning of the section called "The Bearing Capacity Problem" without losing anything critical about the argument. You'll just have to trust me a bit more about some of my claims. Generally speaking, the quality or performance of a health AI system is assessed under one of two different rubrics: agreement and accuracy.[17] Agreement metrics evaluate the extent to which an AI's diagnoses or decisions match the diagnoses or decisions made by the groundtruthing process. An AI with 90% agreement makes the same decision as the groundtruthing process 9 out of 10 times. Accuracy metrics evaluate the extent to which an AI's diagnoses or decisions match the

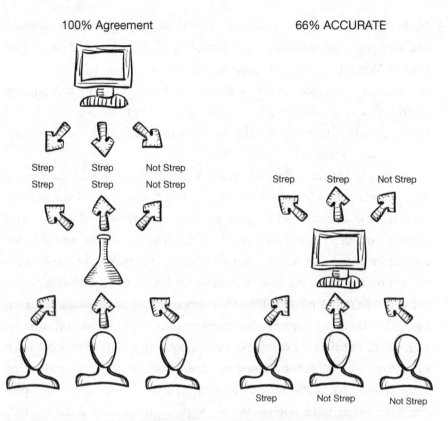

Figure 4.1. AI agreement (right) and accuracy (left) in strep throat diagnostics. Adapted from 0melapics, Set of Hand Drawn Icons, n.d., https://www.freepik.com/free-vector/set-hand-drawn-icons_979925.htm. Public Domain.

actual ground truth. An AI system with an accuracy score of 90% gets the answer right 9 times out of 10.

Figure 4.1 illustrates the difference between agreement and accuracy by imagining an AI system that might try to diagnose strep throat. On the left-hand side, three patients get the usual old-school laboratory test for strep throat. This is an engineered groundtruthing process, and as we know from above, step tests have a sensitivity (correct when positive) of about 86% and a specificity (correct when negative) of around 95%. So, we know the lab test is pretty good, but we know it's not 100% accurate. This means we don't know for sure if any individual patient actually has strep or not. But we can test the agreement between the AI and the strep test.

In this case, it is 100% or perfect agreement. Now, when some researchers test for agreement, they use more complicated measures that correct for chance. When there's only two options (strep vs. not strep), there's a 50% chance that the AI and the lab test agree by luck. The more complicated metrics described in the next section help to filter out this luck factor. Unfortunately, correcting for chance is more common in the social sciences than in health AI.

Moving to accuracy, the right-hand diagram shows three patients with a cough where one (#1 left-to-right) has strep throat. The AI guesses that both the left and the middle patients have strep throat, which makes it right in 2 out of 3 cases or 66% accurate. Accuracy measures mostly do not correct for chance. In fact, percent accuracy (the same percentage of times correct metric I'm using here) is commonly found in the technical literature. As you may already realize, there are a couple of potential problems here. One hundred percent agreement sounds pretty good (and it is for some AIs), but if an AI developer only reports that reliability score (as is often the case), it makes the system seem better than it is at diagnosing strep throat. It's 100% agreement with a known-to-be-imperfect process. The other (and potentially larger problem) is that accuracy tests hide agreement tests. In the right-hand figure, how do we know which patient has strep throat? We only know because a lab test said they do. Despite the term, ground truth is never just there laying on the ground to be seen. Ground truth is always created through a dredging, engineering, or forging process. In this case, it's engineered through a lab test with a known error rate. That lab test has stipulated that patient #1 has strep and the others do not. The stipulative data is the only thing against which we can measure the accuracy of the AI system. That means, essentially, that we are testing agreement with engineered ground truth and calling it accuracy. Accuracy is essentially a special case of reliability where we agree to accept that the results of some groundtruthing process is identical to actual ground truth. This is all the more true in the United States regulatory context. If you read the math details that follow, you'll see that the FDA asks AI manufacturers to calculate agreement or accuracy using the exact same formula. However, they simply ask device manufactures to call the final score something different ("agreement") if the analysis doesn't use certain commonly accepted groundtruthing processes that are assumed to create actual ground truth. (Here's where the math starts, so if you want to skip to the next section, feel free.)

The various metrics just discussed have generally been designed to measure either accuracy or agreement. That is, certain tests are commonly used for accuracy and certain other tests for agreement. Percent accuracy, specificity, sensitivity, and AUC are common accuracy measures, while the various kappas, alphas, and correlation coefficients are statistical measures of agreement. Most agreement and accuracy metrics are calculated based on a confusion matrix, a table detailing the rates of true positives (TP), false positives (FP), true negatives (TN), and false negatives (FN). Table 4.1 provides the formulas for a few of the easier-to-calculate metrics. Metrics like sensitivity and specificity represent certain rates of accuracy, True Positive Rate (TPR) and True Negative Rate (TNR), respectively. Thus, scores are often reported both as either percentages (93.7%) or as decimalized values (.937). These are the same scores, 93.7% = .937. AUC scores are also percentages and thus can also be represented at 82.6% or .826. However, you'll note that I did not include the calculations for AUC in the table. The formula is a mess of derivatives and integrals. While the idea is fairly easy to understand conceptually, it's not an easy math

Table 4.1. SELECTED VALIDITY AND RELIABILITY METRICS

Metric	Purpose	Calculation
Sensitivity, Recall, True Positive Rate (TPR)	Validity	$\dfrac{TP}{TP+FN}$
Specificity, Selectivity, True Negative Rate (TNR)	Validity	$\dfrac{TN}{TP+FN}$
Accuracy	Validity	$\dfrac{TP+TN}{TP+TN+FP+FN}$
Cohen's k	Reliability	$\dfrac{p_o - p_e}{1 - p_e}$

NOTE: p_o = observed agreement or accuracy. p_e = the probability of chance agreement problem. In short, calculating an AUC score is a two-step process. First, you determine the receiver-operating characteristic (ROC) curve, which is essentially a line representing the relationship between the sensitivity and specificity of a binary classifier. Figure 4.2 shows several representative ROC curves. AUC is area under the ROC curve, or the percentage of the chart left in the lower right-hand corner. A perfect classifier (100% sensitivity and specificity) would be two intersecting straight lines that follow the x- and y-axes. A useless classifier (no better than chance) is a straight diagonal line from the lower left corner of the plot to the upper right. The better performing a classifier, the more its ROC curve bends toward the upper left corner, and the more chart area is under the curve: 100% or 1 for a perfect classifier, 50% or .5 for a random classifier, 85% or .85 for an acceptable classifier.

Reliability statistics look a lot like decimalized accuracy scores, and they are certainly similar. It is very common to see articles report κ = .521 or κ = .876. You will basically never see a κ-value represented as a percentage, because the two are not equivalent. A κ-score is a *score* in the truest sense

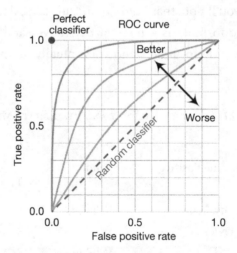

Figure 4.2. Area under the ROC curve examples with guides for qualitative interpretation.
Source: Martin Thoma, Receiver Operating Characteristic (ROC) curve with False Positive Rate and True Positive Rate, 24 June 2018, https://en.wikipedia.org/wiki/Receiver_operating_characteristic#/media/File:Roc-draft-xkcd-style.svg. Public Domain.

of the word. It is a value that has been corrected for chance, rather than an actual percentage. Sometimes, you will see reliability represented by various correlation coefficients. I mentioned Lin's CCC above. The intra-class correlation coefficient (ICC) is also quite common. Correlation coefficients also look the same at first glance, e.g., CCC = .821, but they are the most different. Accuracy statistics and κ-values are on a scale from 0 to 1. Correlation coefficients range from –1 to 1. So, it's possible that a CCC could equal –0.92, which would mean that the raters almost perfectly disagree. They are opposite in each case. Given this morass of similar-looking but not actually equivalent numbers, how does one know when they have a good score? A very good question, without an easy answer.

The creators of accuracy and agreement metrics will largely tell you that it is a mistake to imagine that there is such a thing as a "good" score. These statistics were all designed to make *very specific* comparisons possible. If you have two AI systems that are designed to do the same thing using the same data, you can compare the results using these metrics to figure out which is better. So, if AI #1 has an AUC of 92% and AI #2 has an AUC of 87%, you can say that "AI #1 is more accurate than AI #2." But you aren't really supposed to say, "AI #1 is good," because "good" is highly contextual. Importantly, accuracy and agreement metrics do not help you compare different AI systems designed for different purposes. An AUC of 74% might be perfectly acceptable for Gmail's spam detection algorithm,[18] but not nearly good enough for certain life-and-death medical decisions. Unfortunately, what folks are "supposed to do" with benchmarking metrics is just not what we see in real-world AI development. In fact, there is a whole cottage industry devoted to assigning qualitative evaluations (good, bad, excellent, outstanding) to different scoring thresholds for different metrics. Unfortunately, the available literature also recommends different scoring thresholds for the *same* metrics. As one example, recommendations for interpreting ICCs vary across contexts and disciplines. The threshold of "low" agreement can be from below ICC = 0.40[19] to ICC = 0.50.[20] Fair to moderate agreement thresholds vary the most with recommend ranges from ICC = 0.40 to ICC = 0.75.[21] Most

ICC schemata accept that ICCs greater than 0.60 are fair to good and ICCs greater than 0.75 as good to excellent.

Despite the best recommendations of the statisticians who designed these metrics, it is actually quite easy to Google your way to threshold recommendations. The only real exception is for sensitivity and specificity. Diagnostic medicine is always on the lookout for the best test available. And sometimes, the best test available is not that good. As a result, you tend to see specificity and sensitivity used more comparatively, and there is a real resistance to setting codified thresholds. Nevertheless, it is quite common for researchers to refer to certain values as "low" (e.g., sensitivity = 48%) and certain values as "high" (e.g., specificity = 98%). As such, it is possible to infer loose guidelines for interpreting these scores. Against that aforementioned best advice of statisticians, I, too, will provide some of these guidelines for you in Table 4.2. As you can see, percentage-based scores are fairly comparable in their interpretation. For specificity, sensitivity, and AUC, the scores are generally not described as "good" lower than 90%. Since the calculation for κ-values corrects for chance, the scores are always lower than accuracy metrics that do not. Accordingly, although κ-values look a lot like other scores in format, the interpretive guidelines are much more forgiving. A Cohen's κ of .71 is generally considered a very good score, whereas AUC = .71 is merely "acceptable."

Despite a whole lot of effort devoted to distinguishing between validity and reliability metrics, they are actually quite interoperable. The various metrics (whether optimized for reliability or accuracy) are essentially different ratios of the same confusion matrix values (TP, FP, TN, FN). The differences between them are often more terminological than statistical. As an illustration of this, the FDA's "Statistical Guidance on Reporting Results from Studies Evaluating Diagnostic Tests" addresses the "difference" between accuracy and agreement directly. When a company seeks approval for a new diagnostic test, it must vouch for the test by use of recognized metrics. The FDA allows submitted data to evaluate tests against one of two standards: (1) the reference standard or best available test or (2) a non-reference standard, some other test. A "reference standard" is essentially taken as ground truth, and in this case the FDA

Table 4.2. Selected Guidelines for Interpreting Sensitivity, Specificity, Cohen's κ, and AUC Values

Metric	Qualitative Interpretation
Sensitivity	Low: less than 80%
	Moderate: 80%–89%
	High: 90%–95%
	Very high: greater than 95%
Specificity	Low: less than 80%
	Moderate: 80%–89%
	High: 90%–95%
	Very high: greater than 95%
Cohen's κ[a]	No agreement: 0
	Slight agreement: .01–.20
	Fair agreement: .21–.40
	Moderate agreement: .41–.60
	Substantial: .61–.80
	Almost perfect agreement: .81 or higher
AUC[b]	Poor: less than .7
	Acceptable: .7–.79
	Excellent: .80–.89
	Outstanding: .90 or greater

NOTE: Sensitivity and specificity interpretations are inferred from the literature. Cohen's κ and AUC recommendations are drawn from specific sources cited in the table.

[a] Mary L. McHugh, "Interrater Reliability: The Kapp Statistic," Biochemia Medica 22, no. 3 (2012): 276–282.

[b] Jayawant N. Mandrekar, "Receiver Operating Characteristic Curve in Diagnostic Test Assessment," Journal of Thoracic Oncology 5, no. 9 (2010): 1315–1316.

advises industry to report sensitivity and specificity. However, the FDA also notes that

> When a new test is evaluated by comparison to a non-reference standard, it is impossible to calculate unbiased estimates of sensitivity and specificity . . . . FDA recommends the use of the terms *positive percent agreement* and *negative percent agreement* with the non-reference standard to describe these results.[22]

The phraseology is important here. The FDA directs attention to use the *terms* "positive percent agreement" and "negative percent agreement." The requested statistical calculations are identical to those for specificity and sensitivity. The math behind each metric is outlined in Tables 2 and 3 in the FDA's appendix. As can be seen in each case, the math is identical. Furthermore, as the guidance clearly indicates, "The difference between Table 3 and Table 1 is that the columns of Table 3 do not represent whether the subject has the condition of interest as determined by the reference standard." Interestingly, biomedical journals do not seem to follow this convention. It is relatively common for diagnostic and AI research to use the terms "sensitivity" and "specificity" even when the new system is indexed to a non-reference standard. Essentially, this all means we should understand validity as a special case of reliability where the one labeling process is taken to be ground truth. Even in cases where the underlying calculations for reliability and validity metrics are not the same, they ultimately produce highly similar results. The probability correction in κ and correlation coefficients notwithstanding, reliability metrics and accuracy metrics simply do not measure meaningfully different phenomena. In fact, metrics designed for ostensibly different purposes are highly correlated.[23]

THE BEARING CAPACITY PROBLEM

My Uncle Bill[24] has a pretty cool job. He's a structural engineer for Skidmore, Owings & Merrill. They make tall buildings—*really* tall buildings. I remember him telling me about a sales meeting he had in the early 2000s. Bill goes to these meetings, but as a structural engineer he's not really the "pitch" guy. In any event, I remember him telling me about how the client and the pitch guy kept pushing the proposed building's height up higher and higher until Bill broke out in a cold sweat. About 10 years later, they did the ribbon cutting at Dubai's Burj Khalifa—the tallest building (and the tallest human structure) ever built. It probably goes without saying that a lot goes into building something as tall as the Burj Khalifa (2,722 feet). At that height, engineers not only have to contend with the forces of gravity, but also the regular possibility that the building will be subject to multiple simultaneous weather systems. Keeping the building upright in the face of conflicting geological and meteorological stressors is literally a matter of life and death. To get the job done, Bill invented an entirely new structural engineering system called the "buttressed core." Everybody talks about the buttressed core because it is the cool new invention here. Even *Wired* featured an article on the buttressed core.[25] But, Bill will be the first to tell you that it does not matter how impressive your structural engineering solution is; it won't stand up on a poor foundation. Dubai's soil simply doesn't have the bearing capacity to hold up 2,722 feet and 500,000 metric tons of building without some serious help. So, the Burj Khalifa is built on top of a 3.7-meter-thick concrete "raft," which itself is supported by 192 1.5-meter-thick, 43-meter-deep pilings. In sum, that is 110,000 metric tons of steel and concrete covering 58,900 cubic yards of subterranean space. And that's how you get bearing capacity for a 500,000-ton skyscraper.

DNNs are the buttressed core of AI. They are the cool new engineering innovation that gets all the hype (and all the attention in journal articles, for that matter). And they are cool—no doubt about it. But AI systems built using DNN architectures are only as good as the foundations that support them. Supervised machine learning must be built on a ground truth with sufficient bearing capacity to support the accuracy claims made about the architecture. Since ground truth is always stipulative and can be created through all manner of approaches, this presents a serious concern for deep medicine. How sure can we be that a given groundtruthing exercise creates sufficient bearing capacity? As it turns out, this is one of those cases where we can effectively use AI to study the limits of AI. More specifically, AI allows us to simulate the inaccessible relationship between accuracy and agreement. Figure 4.1 (in the last section) shows the typical frameworks for testing agreement and accuracy. Importantly, when you test accuracy, you assume that the groundtruthing process produced an objective ground truth, so you don't know agreement. In contrast, when you test agreement, you accept that you don't have true ground truth, so you don't know accuracy. The inability to match groundtruthing accuracy directly to AI agreement makes determining the bearing capacity of the groundtruthing process impossible.

Figure 4.2 illustrates what it would take to test the bearing capacity of groundtruthing processes. If we know (1) the actual truth of the patient's status, (2) the best guess of the gold standard lab test, and (3) the best guess of the AI, we could determine the extent to which the lab test is sturdy enough to support an effect strep AI. There is no situation where we could actually know all these values with the possible exception of groundtruth established through subsequent postmortem evaluation. (And this would only work for certain conditions.) Thus, to reliably explore the bearing capacity of ground truth, we must simulate the relationships between an actual ground truth, a lab-test-simulated ground truth, and an AI-generated diagnosis. Thus, in what follows, I present the results of a bearing capacity simulation[26] developed from the canonical Wisconsin Breast Cancer Dataset (WBCD) benchmarking data set.[27] For this simulation, I created 998 cancer diagnostic AI systems in paired sets. The first AI in each pairing stands in for a groundtruthing process with a known accuracy (e.g., a lab test). I created each of these simulated lab tests in such a way that I have accuracy scores that range from essentially no agreement ($\kappa = 0.0356$) to almost perfect agreement ($\kappa = 0.8998$). Using each of the best guesses of each of these simulated lab tests, I trained a second AI to predict whether each patient had cancer or not. This second set of AIs simulates the kinds of diagnostic AIs that were discussed in Chapters 1 and 3. All in all, this simulation allows me to do something that cannot be done in real-world AI development: compare the reportable model accuracy of an AI system based on an engineered ground truth (the hidden reliability in Figure 4.1) to an actual ground truth (true accuracy). Figure 4.3 provides a snapshot of the simulation results.

Ultimately, what this simulation shows us is that the reportable accuracy of diagnostic systems based on engineered ground truth is consistently higher than the actual accuracy of those systems. Differences range from $\kappa = 0.221$ to $\kappa = 0.9259$ with an average of $\kappa = 0.2390$. This magnitude of difference is such that the qualitative description of a system's accuracy will be inflated by at least one level (e.g., fair to moderate or

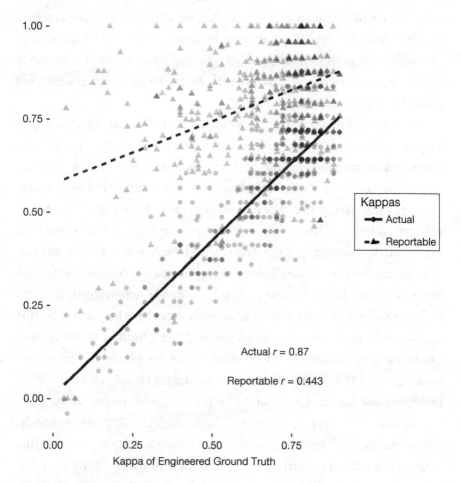

Figure 4.3. Engineered ground truth–bearing capacity simulation.

substantial to almost perfect) in 80.36% of cases. That is, fair agreement would be described as moderate, moderate as substantial, and substantial as almost perfect. Importantly, the magnitude of the difference reliably increases as the performance of the engineered ground truth degrades. Bearing capacity falls off significantly below $\kappa = 0.7$. Based on this simulation, you would need an engineered ground truth of $\kappa \geq 0.75$ to be fairly confident that the final system performance was more than moderate ($\kappa > 0.6$). Of course, there are more than a few published AI systems built on engineered ground truth accuracies of 0.6 or lower. Finally, the correlation values (r) reported in Figure 4.3 show us that while the underlying theory of benchmarking is sound (actual accuracy correlates very strongly with the accuracy of engineered ground truth), the common practice is significantly flawed. It is typically only possible to report accuracy values based on engineered ground truth's predictions, and those reportable accuracy values do not correlate as strongly with actual accuracy when measured against true ground truth.

This simulation also raises questions about the bearing capacity of forged ground truth. To explore this question, I created consensus-based recommendations for 200 random pairings of the original simulated lab tests described above.[28] I then compared the agreement of each paring with the overall accuracy of the consensus-based recommendations. The results are available in Figure 4.4. As was the case with the forged ground truth simulation, these results suggest that the underlying theory behind using forged approaches to ground truth is sound. However, the practical guidance regarding sufficiently high agreement is again out of sync with actual performance. In this case as well, agreement scores of $\kappa > 0.75$ are required to more than moderate final model accuracy. Again, there are plenty of consensus-based ground truth agreement scores in the literature where $\kappa < 0.75$, including notably the CCC[29] of 0.35 reported above. Importantly, some low agreement scores ($\kappa = .55$) had high accuracy ($\kappa = .8$), but additional efforts are likely needed to assure system accuracy. And, this leads to the critical importance of "platinum standard" AI, which I discuss in the next section.

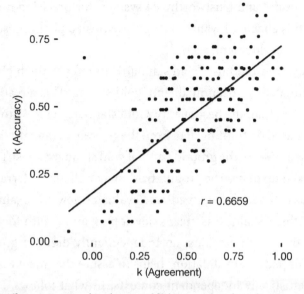

Figure 4.4. Difference in actual and reportable kappa values based on known accuracy of engineered ground truth.

PLATINUM STANDARD AI

Over the course of this chapter, I have explored several uncomfortable facts about AI development: (1) Many approaches to groundtruthing are deeply problematic. Dredged and engineered ground truth is subject to all sorts of systemic and availability biases, and forged ground truth frequently masks its limitations through single-rater designs, hierarchical rating teams, or overly large rating teams. (2) The rhetoric of validity metrics imagines that they are substantively different from agreement metrics, when the difference is merely a questionable stipulation of ground truth. (3) The bearing capacity problem exposes a serious likelihood that many AI development teams are significantly overstating the accuracy of the systems they design. Based on the simulations described previously, both engineered and forged ground truth designs require higher baseline metrics than often appear in the published literature in order to assure reasonably performant systems. Taken together, one might infer that I think all AI is hype. This isn't the case at all. Rather, I think it is quite possible to develop useful and trustworthy AI systems for precision medicine. So, in closing this chapter, I want to reflect briefly on a platinum standard example of AI development.

Normally, we would use "gold standard" to refer to the highest quality, but unfortunately, in deep medicine "gold standard" is already taken for something less than the best quality. Gold standard AI is AI that has been developed based on training data from the reference standard. However, as we have already seen, the ground truth of gold standard AI isn't necessarily all it's cracked up to be. The ground truth may well not be terra firma after all. Platinum standard deep medicine evaluates new AIs against multiple ground truths. Usually, this means developing an AI with forged ground truth and then testing against an independently dredged ground truth. This form of "external validation" helps to assure that the AI is reliable in multiple statistically independent contexts. In what follows, I briefly describe an ideal illustration of the platinum standard in the development of an AI system designed to help diagnose intracranial hemorrhage.

Accurately diagnosing the nature and extent of head injuries is a common problem in emergency rooms and trauma centers. Motor vehicle accidents, falls, violence, and child abuse are the most common causes of head trauma and can lead to all manner of serious injury and even death. One particular injury that trauma doctors are always on the lookout for is the intracranial hemorrhage. Ruptured or leaky blood vessels in the skull can cause blood to pool and lead to increased intracranial pressure, potentially crushing delicate brain matter. In a trauma setting, a computed tomography scan (CT scan or CAT scan) is the go-to option for diagnosing intracranial hemorrhage. As discussed in previous chapters, radiology is as much art as science. Reading X-rays, CT scans, MRIs, etc., requires years of training and experience. As a result, medical science is increasingly looking toward AI to improve the accuracy of imaging-based diagnoses.

One promising new AI in this area uses deep convolutional neural networks (DCNNs) to diagnose intracranial hemorrhage from CT scans. The results of the benchmarking study are described in an article published in the journal *Nature Biomedical Engineering*.[30] As the paper describes, engineered groundtruthing was implemented by a non-hierarchical team of "five subspecialty-trained US board-certified neuroradiologists."[31] Given the high levels of training, the non-hierarchical team structure, and the fact that five is on the bubble before the paradox of unanimity starts becoming a problem, this is likely a very good approximation of actual ground truth. The team trained four different DCNN architectures in order to develop an ensemble model with a very high AUC score of 0.99. Importantly, the study reports the precision rates of each individual model and the ensemble. Up to this point, I might describe this study as compelling and well executed. What really makes its approach "platinum standard" is the quality of its external validity assessments.

Much of AI is developed solely based on *internal* validity. Internal validity is determined by taking a groundtruthed data set and cutting it up into training and validation sets. A development team might groundtruth 500 cases, using 300 to train and 200 to validate. External validity involves measuring the AI system against another data set, unrelated to the training and validation sets. The intracranial hemorrhage diagnostic AI offers an especially impressive approach to external validity. Initial training and internal validation were based on a retrospective study. That is, the researchers collected CT scans from patient charts, and the groundtruthing team labeled them for AI training and testing. Once this process was complete, the research team also collected a prospective data set. That is, they investigated CT scan records from patients admitted after the development of the new system. Importantly, the prospective/external validity set was groundtruthed by a different team of radiologists not privy to the study design or AI architecture. Here the article reports groundtruthing interrater reliability: "The agreements between the radiologists were 94% (radiologists A and B), 93% (radiologists B and C) and 90% (radiologists A and C)."[32] It also reports agreement with the AI system: "The agreements between 3 independent neuroradiologists and the algorithm for selecting morphologically similar prediction-basis images were 93%, 94% and 95%, with Cohen's kappa values of 0.91, 0.92 and 0.93, respectively."[33] Ultimately, the ensemble model demonstrated an impressive AUC of 0.96 against the prospective test set.

It is this high degree of triangulation that makes these data so compelling. "Triangulation" is a nautical metaphor. If you do not quite know where you are at sea, you can determine your position by getting bearings (compass readings) on three or more fixed points on land. With only one bearing, you only know yourself to be along a straight line. Two bearings provide an approximation. The more bearings you have, the more precisely you can calculate your position. Essentially the same holds true for groundtruthing and AI system accuracy. A single-rater design is unreliable because you only have one point of reference. A robust, non-hierarchical, independent groundtruthing with proper agreement does a better job of "fixing" ground truth. Multi-model triangulation as part of ensembling and robust multi-vector external validity assessments all contribute to a more compelling case for the accuracy and utility of a new AI system.

Failure to validate externally a new AI system can lead to some embarrassing and dangerous outcomes. Recently a research team at the University of Michigan found that a widely used model for sepsis prediction performed much more poorly than originally advertised.[34] Epic is one of the largest providers of EMR systems in use, and its proprietary Epic Sepsis Model was marketed based on internal validity benchmarks ranging from AUC = 0.76 to AUC = 0.83. Importantly, the Epic Sepsis Model was trained on a proxy measure, *International Statistical Classification of Diseases and Related Health Problems* (ICD) billing codes for sepsis. Unfortunately, billing codes are unreliable proxies for sepsis. Karandeep Singh and his team at the University of Michigan conducted their own external validity study of the sepsis model and found that the true system performance was closer to AUC = 0.63.[35] Ultimately, this case points to serious risks of early adoption for sub-platinum-standard systems.

To make matters worse, even though platinum standard methods are readily available and widely known, they are unfortunately not the most common. A recent meta-study, designed to assess the extent to which diagnostic AI really was as accurate as human doctors, evaluated 82 studies for methodological quality.[36] The meta-study authors lamented that "a major finding of the review is that few studies presented externally validated results or compared the performance of deep learning models and health-care professionals using the same sample."[37] While 76 (93%) of the studies used gold standard methods, only 29 (35%) used a platinum standard approach.[38] Interestingly, the meta-study still ultimately concluded that diagnostic health AI was "equivalent to that of health-care professionals."[39] The seeming contradiction in these findings is what most concerns my work in this book. If a study uses a less-than-platinum-standard approach, in the face of many known issues with groundtruthing, then how can one conclude that the AI system is "equivalent" to health-care professionals? The gap between evidentiary foundation and accuracy claims is the literal locus of hype and the primary concern of *The Doctor and the Algorithm.*

Thus, in the next chapter, I turn to a counterdata-inspired exercise, one designed to understand better the nature and prevalence of hype in deep medicine. Chapter 5 proceeds in two parts: The first offers textual analyses of hype in medical futurism, press releases, biomedical journal articles, and the news media. These analyses show how the most extravagant claims about the potential of deep medicine persist across a wide range of publication venues. The second part of Chapter 5 reports on my development and uses an AI system that identifies and classifies promotional language in biomedical research. With this system, I explore the extent of promotional language in a sample of 973 health AI articles published in 319 journals between 2019 and 2021. Additionally, by comparing the distribution of promotional language to information on the quality of a subset of the underlying studies, I can start to shed real light on the prevalence of hype in scientific research on deep medicine.

HypeDx

"[A]rtificial intelligence" has been burdened with meaning by marketing hype, popular culture, and science fiction—possibly impeding a reasoned and balanced discourse.

—*Artificial Intelligence in Health Care: The Hope, the Hype, the Promise, the Peril.*[1]

The epigraph above comes from a recent National Academy of Medicine report on health AI. While the report title centers concerns about hype, hype—itself—is actually not much discussed in the 269 pages. Where hype is engaged, it is described in terms much like the above. That is, hype is assumed to be a feature of anything other than the science itself. Hype comes from marketing, pop culture, and science fiction, but not from biomedical research. Within this context, the overwhelming drive of the report is to navigate safely Gartner's "hype cycle," which describes the popular reception of new technology as a progression through four phases: the peak of inflated expectations, the trough of disillusionment, the slope of enlightenment, and the plateau of productivity. According to the report authors, this path to technological "maturity" is fraught because "Without an appreciation for both the capabilities and limitations

The Doctor and the Algorithm. S. Scott Graham, Oxford University Press. © Oxford University Press 2022.
DOI: 10.1093/oso/9780197644461.003.0006

of AI technology in medicine, we will predictably crash into a 'trough of disillusionment.' The greatest risk of all may be such a backlash that impedes real progress toward using AI tools to improve human lives."[2] In describing how best to avert this risk, they further argue that "explicit advertising hyperbole may be one of the most direct triggers for unintended consequences of hype," and that "A combination of technical and subject domain expertise is needed to recognize the credible potential of AI systems and avoid the backlash that will come from overselling them."[3]

Ultimately, the National Academy of Medicine's analysis replicates the long-discredited two-stage model of dissemination and popularization where, as Stephen Hilgartner puts it, "first, scientists develop genuine scientific knowledge; subsequently, popularizers disseminate simplified accounts to the public."[4] The report assumes that good science happens first, and that hyperbole largely arises only when that good science is tainted by profit motive and redeployed as a part of advertising and promotional efforts. Unfortunately, this conception is often shared by researchers who wish to understand the nature and distribution of hype in scientific and biomedical research. In recent years, there have been several projects devoted to identifying hype in science writing. These projects typically aim to develop methods and approaches that can reliably identify exaggeration in popular news media. In so doing, researchers generally compare the claims of scientific journal articles to related claims in popular media. Any evidence of mismatch is assumed to be the media's bastardization of good science. For example, Li, Zhang, and Yu trained a support vector machine (SVM) using a data set of paired scientific journal and news articles annotated for claim strength.[5] That is, they taught an AI to look for textual markers of exaggeration in paired scientific and media claims. Where the media exaggeration was greater, hype was assumed. Similarly, Patro and Burah used a word-embedding model to evaluate claim strength and compute the difference between paired claims in the scientific literature and popular press.[6] In another example, Yu, Wang, Guo, and Li developed a machine-learning system that identified hype in press releases based on a mismatch between associative statistical tests and causal claims.[7] If the scientific study merely tested for correlation, but the media article described that association in terms of causality, hype was assumed. By-and-large, this kind of research rests on the assumption that hype happens at the stage of popularization and not in the scientific literature itself. In so doing, these studies (1) embrace the two-stage model, (2) assume that claims in scientific journals are accurate and unbiased, and (3) interpret any deviation in the popular media as a result of sensationalization.

In the past several chapters, I have been working against this limited conception of hype. In Chapter 3, I described health AI's integrated marcom framework—the closely linked promotional initiatives of scientific publications, press releases, and marketing materials. The analysis of iCAD's marcom strategy for the ProFound AI™ system shows how closely connected promotional efforts in scientific and nonscientific venues can be. Additionally, Chapter 4 showcases the limits of some groundtruthing approaches and highlights how scientific research can be misled by incorrect assumptions about a ground truth's bearing capacity. In cases where the groundtruthing approach is problematic and external validation is lacking, strong claims about system performance in the biomedical literature are highly likely to be hype. So, in continuing these lines of inquiry, the overarching goal of this chapter is to get a better handle on the true extent of hype in scientific publications about health AI. Subsequently, I describe the development and application of the HypeDx system, a binary classifier that can identify promotional language in technical abstracts. However, before I dive into this analysis, there is more to say about the root of hype across marcom networks. While the two-stage model is fatally flawed, this certainly does not mean that PR and media accounts of deep medicine are without hype. Rather, they are frequently hyperbolic, but often in ways that can be traced back to the original scientific publications or authors. Thus, before turning to the HypeDx system I begin with a brief exploration of hype as it circulates through the various genres of marcom networks.

THE ROOT OF HYPE

The problematic two-stage model of popularization often focuses on a dichotomy between the idealized presentation of information in scientific reports and media reports. Analyses built on this dichotomy often miss out on a critical intermediary genre—the press release. In a fiercely competitive media economy, attracting journalistic attention is no easy task. Science journalists often do not have the time to leisurely browse the roughly 2.6 million scientific articles published every year. Thus, the press release and the online aggregator have become critical resources for attracting media attention. EurekAlert! is a press release aggregator sponsored by the American Academy for the Advancement of Science (AAAS). PR professionals at universities, in industry, and at various research nonprofits use this aggregator, in addition to many others, to try to reach a broader public audience. Press releases (on EurekAlert! and elsewhere) typically offer a concise (300–400 word) summary of recent scientific findings. Such press releases have been regularly criticized for exaggerating the significance of new findings, and EurekAlert!, in particular, insofar as it bares the prestigious AAAS imprint, has been asked to consider more aggressive approaches to moderation.[8] Nevertheless, a hasty search of EurekAlert! shows that, as expected, extravagant language remains stock-in-trade in press releases about health AI.

When searching for "health AI," the first results (as of the day of this writing) all point toward speed, accuracy, overcoming bias, and reducing the costs of care. The media relations team at Northwestern University in Chicago posted a EurekAlert! press release in May 2020 that artfully illustrates typical appeals to AI speed. "Northwestern University researchers are using artificial intelligence (AI) to speed up the search for COVID-19 treatments and vaccines. The AI-powered tool makes it possible to prioritize resources for the most promising studies—and ignore research that is unlikely to yield benefits."[9] Likewise, an August 2020 release from the technology company Babylon demonstrates a standard appeal to increased accuracy:

Dr Jonathan Richens, Babylon scientist and lead author, said: "We took an AI with a powerful algorithm, and gave it the ability to imagine alternate realities and consider 'would this symptom be present if it was a different disease'? This allows the AI to tease apart the potential causes of a patient's illness and score more highly than over 70% of the doctors on these written test cases."[10]

Although speed and accuracy are usually among the most popular claims about AI, another very common one is cost savings. A 2016 Binghamton University press release promises a data-driven algorithmic solution that will reduce inefficiencies in pharmacy management and "save money."[11] And not for nothing, the same press release also appeals to a long-standing clinical bugbear—the so-called problem of patient compliance. Quoting the project lead, Sang Won Yoon, the press release suggests potential in this area: "Additionally, we can apply this research to both enhance pharmacy automation and management, and to help us understand patients' medication adherence and compliance issues in the future."[12]

For the trifecta of what are probably the most common promotional claims, the research nonprofit eLife issued a press release in November 2020 touting a new system that "speeds up biology and removes potential human bias."[13] Here, the headline justifies the accuracy claim by referencing the common failures of human psychology. Interestingly, the body text of this press release does not actually address "bias" in any way. Of course, none of this should be surprising. The press release phase of a marcom strategy is exactly where we would expect to find hype. Nevertheless, its position as a medial element between publication and popularization and the fact that many of them are written by researchers themselves do much to dismantle the presuppositions of the two-stage model. What's more, as it turns out, scientific press releases might actually be more prone to hype than press releases from other sectors. According to one analysis of press releases and their broader circulation in the media, biomedical and scientific PR exists at a point of significant tension between promotional and educational demands.[14] Effective science PR must present the sponsoring institution in a good light, explain novel scientific processes to public audiences, and grab the attention of journalists. The conflict be-tween these demands "creates a tension as the goal of journalistic attention depends on hype or some other link to public values and interests that po-tentially stand in contrast to a faithful representation of the science."[15] This tension all but requires hype for resolution. The "boring" didactic content of scientific education must be counterbalanced with promotional lan-guage that garners journalistic attention and investment. As Lynch et al. further explain,

> [I]f the scientific vision dominates, then the story might fail to draw the attention of journalists. In other words, PR practitioners working in biomedical research settings face con-flicting demands: As they attempt to promote the organization's accomplishments, one audience demands they explain or teach the science, while the other wants relevant and newsworthy stories brought to their attention.[16]

If hype is a feature, not a bug, of PR and the press release, where does that leave us? Where do we go for measured information about deep med-icine? Perhaps, the editorial standards of popular news media and aca-demic journals limit the propensity for hype.[17]

The promotional language we find in press releases is plenty preva-lent in science journalism. Indeed, it is not difficult to find the standard tropes of speed, accuracy, and the like. A 2018 *Harvard Business Review* article asks patients to get over their skepticism about health AI because "it can perform with expert-level accuracy and deliver cost-effective care at scale."[18] In *Business Insider*, we can read about how Google Health's DeepMind AI "can outperform doctors on identifying breast cancer from X-ray images."[19] Likewise, the *New York Times* tells us that "The ability to process vast amounts of data may make it possible for artificial intelli-gence to recognize subtle patterns that humans [doctors] simply cannot see."[20] I have focused a lot on diagnostic applications of AI because the language of "outperformance" makes it easy to see the promotional ele-ment. However, one of the most enduring areas of health AI enthusiasm centers around the hope that it will free physicians from the shackles of data entry. Per *FastCompany*,

> Doctors also spend an enormous amount of time entering data in the electronic health record. Ku says that doctors have what's called "pajama time," which refers to the hours they spend at home recalling patient information into the system. This is why doctors would love a notetaking experience that was more akin to talking to Alexa.[21]

All-in-all, hype appears alive and well in the news media.

While one might have expected that journalistic and editorial practices would make reporting on innovations in health AI more immune to hype, this is not the case. This situation is due, in no small part, to the fact that press releases are often adopted word for word as news articles. The aforementioned analysis of press releases and subsequent media distribution found that

> Within the journalistic coverage as a whole (i.e., duplicate, refashioned, and new articles), institutional press release material makes up the bulk of the content, and new material constitutes less than 40% of the entire article (Table 3). When examining only stories coded as "new" journalistic articles, institutional PR, along with a small contribution from third-party PR material, makes up 40% of the total article. The material from institutional press releases is equally presented verbatim and paraphrased in all stories, but "new" articles favor paraphrasing (Table 4).[22]

It is worth noting that this kind of direct appropriation may not be uniform across news outlets. There's good reason to believe that prestige outlets that tend to have designated science journalists on staff (*New York Times, Washington Post, BBC*) are less likely to appropriate whole passages from press releases.

While the promotional efforts of institutional press releases are often blamed for the extravagant language that finds its way into the media, a recent BBC article ("AI 'outperforms' doctors diagnosing breast cancer"[23]) offers an interesting case where the journal article, itself, is actually more promotional than the corresponding press release. The abstract of the original *Nature* reporting on this particular AI system is quick to declare, "Here we present an artificial intelligence (AI) system that is capable of surpassing human experts in breast cancer prediction."[24] In contrast, the more measured press release from the PR team at the Imperial College of London only states that "The findings, published in *Nature*, show the AI was able to correctly identify cancers from the images with a similar degree of accuracy to expert radiologists, and holds the potential to assist clinical staff in practice."[25] Now, the promotional language of the media coverage in this case did catch some blowback. It is possible that the press release's language was moderated after the fact. Yet, the Internet Archive shows this language dating back to the first snapshot on January 6, 2020, only a few days after *Nature* published the original article. Regardless of the specific pedigree here, it is clear promotional language is alive and well in biomedical publishing.

Ultimately, it does not take long to find scholarly research articles that trot out the same talking points about speed, accuracy, and bias. Becker et al.'s deep learning mammography toolkit "learns better and faster than a human reader with no prior experience."[26] The onychomycosis diagnostic system discussed in Chapter 3 "precisely matched the test data sets from three different sources."[27] And, a recent article from *JAMA Ophthalmology* hits most of the standard hype talking points before offering a new twist on AI's potential to overcome bias:

> The i-ROP DL algorithm outperformed not only most experts in this study but also all prior [computer-based image analysis] systems. . . . [O]ur current system performed almost perfectly and performed better than most experts on the test set of 100 images at 3-level diagnosis (normal vs pre–plus disease vs plus disease) using raw image files without the need for manual segmentation. We also observed that each of the experts' operating points for sensitivity and specificity of diagnosis of plus disease fell on or near the ROC

curve for the DL algorithm, suggesting that the diagnosis of individual experts may be predicted by tuning the operating point and/or slightly retraining the CNN to better understand that expert's unique biases.[28]

Here, the authors suggest that i-ROP DL could be used not only to diagnose retinopathy, but also to diagnose clinical biases. Through tuning the algorithm to mimic individual biases, those biases might be exposed and corrected.

All in all, these examples show how hype in original scientific articles can feed into media ecologies either directly or through marcom efforts and related press releases. Once again, we have more evidence that the two-stage model of scientific popularization is fatally flawed. But importantly, *can* is not the same thing as *does regularly*. In the last few pages, I have presented a handful of carefully curated examples of hype in scientific articles, related press releases, and follow-up media coverage. While these examples showcase the limits of the two-stage model, they do not offer any evidence about the true distribution of hype in biomedical publishing on health AI. This is a question that is well worth addressing. Hype may be rare. It may be common. Figuring out which is the case is a critical component of guiding efforts to separate the promise from the peril in deep medicine. Thus, in what follows, I outline my own counterdata-inspired exercise designed to address just this question.

A COUNTERDATA-INSPIRED EXERCISE

In Donna Haraway's famous *Modest. Witness*, she invokes the figure of the gynecological speculum to explain the value of "diffractive" research methodologies. Haraway's metaphor of diffraction is based on what happens when white light passes through a prism. The many wavelengths that make up the light are diffracted, and the constituent parts (red, orange, yellow, green, blue, and violet) are exposed. As she argues, diffractive or feminist, antiracist, and emancipatory research practices are those that open up occluded spaces to view. They showcase the machinations of power and the effects those machinations have on marginalized peoples. Although her diffractive method is deeply indebted to a critical epistemological framework that rejects the supposed apolitical and objective nature of science, Haraway is more than willing to make use of the techniques of objectivity if doing so serves emancipatory ends. As she notes,

> A speculum does not have to be a literal physical tool for prying open tight orifices; it can be any instrument for rendering a part accessible to observation. So, I will turn to another kind of speculum—statistical analysis coupled with freedom- and justice-oriented policy formation . . . [29]

For Haraway, feminist, antiracist, and emancipatory statistics are entirely continuous with her critical feminist methodology. As she goes on to argue,

> In Theodore Potter's terms (1994; 1995), statistics is a basic technology for crafting objectivity and stabilizing facts. Objectivity is less about realism than it is about intersubjectivity. The impersonality of statistics is one aspect of the complex intersubjectivity of objectivity; that is, of the public quality of technical scientific knowledge. Feminists have high stakes in the speculum of statistical knowledge for opening up otherwise invisible, singular experience to reconfigure public, widely lived reality.[30]

Echoing this sentiment, Catherine D'Ignazio and Lauren Klein's Data Feminism notes that "Data are part of the problem, to be sure. But they are also part of the solution."[31] Effectively, marshaled data can disrupt and diffract (to use Haraway's term) notions of objectivity and authority in powerful systems.

In outlining ways that data can be part of the solution, they focus primarily on what they call "counterdata." Counterdata, in a data feminism idiom, generally has two primary features: (1) it is justice oriented, that is, collected expressively for the purposes of intervening in systems of power and oppression, and (2) it is usually collected by the communities most affected by systemic injustice. A primary example from the text is Mariá Sagulero's collection of "a comprehensive dataset on femicides—gender-related killings of women and girls" in Mexico.[32] Counterdata is frequently about documenting the undocumented. Whereas the Mexican government is not systematically tracking femicide nationally, Sagulero steps in to draw attention to the issue. The data exercise I offer here is inspired both by Haraway's notion of diffractive specula and D'Ignazio and Klein's attention to counterdata. Importantly, *inspired* is the key term here. This exercise is not quite counterdata. It aims at providing occluded data to intervene in processes that often lead to marginalization, but the data are not generated by the most affected community members. However, given all these issues with typical groundtruthing practices (as described in the last chapter), it strikes me as very much worth the effort of trying to render visible just how much researchers might be overstating the accuracy of precision medicine.

HYPEDX

In order to evaluate the extent of hype in deep medicine, I developed the HypeDx AI system, a classifier that can identify promotional language in abstracts from health AI publications. The overall approach to groundtruthing would qualify as forged under the criteria set forth in Chapter 4. The development of the HypeDx system and the subsequent analyses rely on several different data sets. In order to avoid confusion, I'm going to describe each of those data sets here first before I move on to a more detailed description of the methods and results. As Table 5.1 indicates, the work of this chapter is built on three different data sets: a training data set, a primary data set of the 973 relevant articles drawn from PubMed, and a random sample of 98 extracted from the 973. The Training Set was used to train the HypeDx AI. The primary AI-driven analysis is based on the PubMed-973 data set, and I also conducted several more fine-grained human-driven analyses on the abstracts in Random-98.

Table 5.1. DATA SETS USED IN HYPEDX DEVELOPMENT AND ANALYSES

Data Set	N of Abstracts	Source
Training Set	82	Articles reviewed in a previously published meta-study of health AI.[a]
PubMed-973	973	PubMed search
Random-98	98	Random sample of 100 PubMed-973 articles, with two exclusions

[a] Liu et al., "A Comparison."

As indicated in Table 5.1, the Training Set was drawn from 82 articles analyzed in a preexisting meta-study of AI performance.[33] In order to evaluate the distribution of hype, I cut the collected abstracts up into 922 individual sentences. Each of these sentences was annotated by two research assistants for evidence of promotional language about developed AI system(s). A given sentence was classified as promotional when one of the following was present: (1) favorable comparisons to human raters or previously developed health ML systems, (2) superlative qualifying adjectives describing the performance or efficiency of the system, (3) claims to generalizability or clinical applicability, or (4) assertions that system performance meets the standards for FDA clearance or approval. I developed this taxonomy of promotional language markers based on a more inductive and rhetorically grounded analysis of selected abstracts and in consultation with the literature on typical genre features of biomedical abstracts (about which, more to be discussed below). Importantly, in this taxonomy, a given sentence was only annotated as "promotional language" if it described a system under evaluation in the article. Promotional language about AI, in general, was not assigned to the "promotional" category. Additionally, claims about system performance that might be considered objectively good (e.g., AUC = .9997) were not classified as "promotional" unless the sentence also included favorable comparisons, superlative qualifiers, claims to generalizability/applicability, or claims to meeting regulatory standards. Further details about these features and illustrative examples are available in Table 5.2 and in the Technical Appendix (section A.2.1). Interrater reliability was almost perfect ($\kappa = 0.825$ with a 94.5%

agreement), and I reconciled any disagreements between raters before training the model.

Just as was the case with the health AI systems in preceding chapters, linguistic data needs to be quantitized through some feature engineering process before it can be submitted to modeling. For HypeDx, I used an approach I developed called Parts-of-Speech average location (POS aveloc). I designed POS aveloc specifically for use in computational rhetoric.[34] POS aveloc quantitizes each sentence based on the average location of each part of speech. It works well for situations where (1) the unit of analysis is a sentence, (2) the collected sentences are fairly homogeneous in terms of content, and (3) the label of interest is a rhetorical or linguistic strategy. POS aveloc features were submitted to a Bagged Classification and Regression Tree (CART) model, and the resulting system has a reportable AUC of 0.8947 or excellent approaching outstanding.[35] Given the insights of the bearing capacity simulations in Chapter 4, we cannot take this score at face value. However, since the underlying interrater reliability was so high, it is unlikely that the true performance would degrade enough to result in a lower qualitative interpretation.

With a functional HypeDx, I was ready to find out just how common hype is in health AI. The next step was to download the abstracts for 1,000 relevant research articles. To do so, I searched PubMed (the U.S. National Library of Medicine's database of than 32 million publications in the biological and biomedical sciences) for "machine learning[MeSH Terms]) AND (AUC[Title/Abstract] OR AUROC[Title/Abstract]." The structure of this search query tells PubMed to find results that include publications classified as "machine learning" according to the Medical Subject Headings (MeSH) ontology and that mentioned AUC or AUROC in the title or abstract. This last parameter helped ensure that the bulk of the results would be for articles that evaluated the performance of one or more specific health AI systems. After collecting the initial 1,000 results, I excluded records for review articles, meta-studies, comments, and other non-research article genres. After removing hits for articles in languages other than English, I was left with 973 health AI articles (hence, PubMed-973) published in 319 journals between 2019 and 2021. The most

Table 5.2. COMMON FEATURES OF PROMOTIONAL LANGUAGE AND EXAMPLES

Promotional Feature	Description and Examples
Favorable Comparison	Sentence asserts that an ML system performs as well as or better than a qualified medical expert or previously developed ML system. • For the first time, dermatologist-level image classification was achieved on a clinical image classification task without training on clinical images. • For the whole-slide image classification task, the best algorithm (AUC, 0.994 [95% CI, 0.983–0.999]) performed significantly better than the pathologists WTC in a diagnostic simulation (mean AUC, 0.810 [range, 0.738–0.884]; $P < .001$).
Superlative Qualifier	Sentence uses positive-valence superlative adjectives or adverbs to qualify claim. • The significant improvements in diagnostic accuracy that we observed in this study show that deep learning methods are a mechanism by which senior medical specialists can deliver their expertise to generalists on the front lines of medicine, thereby providing substantial improvements to patient care. • Further, RADnet achieves higher recall than two of the three radiologists, which is remarkable.
Generalizability or Applicability	Sentence claims that findings are generalizable or warrant use in clinical contexts. • These methods could be of benefit to centers at which thoracic imaging expertise is scarce, as well as for stratification of patients in clinical trials. • Collectively, the current system may have capabilities for screening purposes in general medical practice, particularly because it requires only a single clinical image for classification.

(*continued*)

Table 5.2. CONTINUED

Promotional Feature	Description and Examples
Regulatory Standards	Sentence asserts that findings meet standards for regulatory approval (e.g., superior or noninferior).

- The three-dimensional convolutional neural network described in this article demonstrated both high sensitivity and high specificity in classifying pulmonary nodules regardless of diameters as well as superiority compared with manual assessment.
- The sensitivity of the DL algorithm for diagnosing ONFH using digital radiography was noninferior to that of both less experienced and experienced radiologist assessments.

common journals were *Scientific Reports*, *PloS One*, the *European Journal of Radiology*, the *Proceedings of the Annual International Conference of the IEEE Engineering in Medicine and Biology Society*, and *BMC Medical Informatics and Decision Making*. Each of these journals was represented between 26 and 99 times.

Once I had the PubMed-973 in hand, I cut up the new abstracts by sentence and used POS aveloc to extract features. HypeDx identified between 0 and 17 promotional sentences per abstract (mean 2.93). The least promotional abstract was 0% promotional and the most promotional abstract was 68.42% promotional. On average, collected abstracts were 23.79% promotional. Genre analysts John Swales and Christine Feak identify five primary discursive moves that are present in most abstracts: (1) background/introduction/situation, (2) present research / purpose, (3) methods/material/subjects/procedures, (4) results/findings, and (5) discussion/conclusion/implications/recommendations.[36] As Swales and Feak indicate, move 5 is the typical location for promotional language, and a certain amount of such language is expected in all abstracts, especially in biomedical science and engineering contexts. Importantly, however, move 5 also tends to be a fairly small portion of the overall abstract. Based on the examples provided by Swales and Feak, typical abstracts devote about 20% of sentences to move 5. While HypeDx does not assess the five moves, it does identify promotional language (which is common to move 5). Since this data set includes 23.79% promotional language, it is likely to be representative of abstracts in general. With Swales and Feak's generic analysis of abstracts as a guide, it is possible to identify provisional guidelines for hype (excessive promotion). Abstracts that devote more than 20% of sentences to promotional language are at moderate risk of hype, and abstracts with more than 40% promotional language (or double the generic standard) are at high risk of hype. Using these thresholds as a guide, Figure 5.1 shows the number of abstracts in each hype risk band. According to this analysis, 393 (40.4%) of the collected articles are at a low risk of hype; 506 (52%) are at a moderate risk of hype; and 74 (7.61%) are at a high risk of hype. Of, course, hype is not necessarily just a matter of promotional language rates. It's also a question of the differential between the underlying quality of the research and the language used to describe that research. Superlative language about a high-performing AI system might not necessarily be "hype." Thus, in the next analysis, I consider what it might mean to correct for underlying system performance in hype analysis.

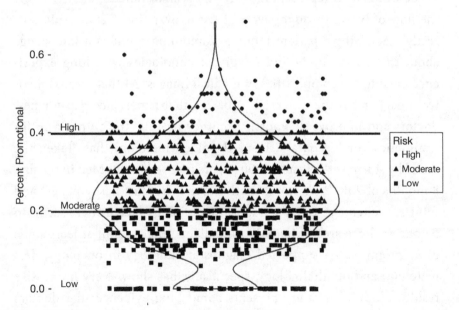

Figure 5.1. Hype risk bands based on abstract conventions.

PERFORMANCE-CORRECTED HYPEDX

Clinical decision support systems or expert systems aim to improve care overall by augmenting human medical decision-making with AI insights. The architects of expert systems intend to support the full continuum of care by improving diagnosis, shaping treatment decisions, and evaluating patient outcomes. Errors in medical decision-making are more common than most people realize, and expert systems are often touted as one way of reducing error rates: "Medical errors are common and costly and can result in death and serious injury. . . . [Expert systems] can aid at building a safer health by providing more precise diagnosis and a more scientific determination of the treatment plan . . . "[37] This is a common trope among AI enthusiasts. Humans make mistakes. Computers might help them make fewer. Of particular attention in deep medicine has been the drive to improve diagnostic accuracy. For example, one of the most active areas of AI development is in diagnostic radiology. Reading an X-Ray or a CT scan is part art and part science. Many cutting-edge radiology technologies collapse 4D data onto a 2D representation. A PET scan or functional MRI shows the flow of blood through layers of tissue over time. As a result, correctly diagnosing a patient requires combining significant knowledge about the human body and imaging technologies with long experience parsing the complexities of medical images. AI that "reads" medical imaging has the potential to bridge that experience gap for new doctors and improve diagnostic accuracy overall. The enthusiasm for "radiomics," or big data–driven AI-guided radiology, has "taken the world by storm with close to 1000 papers indexed in PubMed in the first 8 months of 2019."[38] Research in this area is not just flashy papers and futurist excitement. In fact, diagnostic radiology increasingly seems to be one of those areas where deep medicine might fulfill at least some of its promises. AI-supported diagnostic radiology in oncology, dermatology, and ophthalmology, specifically, has shown very impressive results. Study after study presents compelling evidence that doctors working with AI are more likely to diagnose correctly certain tumors, skin ailments, and eye conditions.

Given the impressive performance of some areas of AI like radiomics, the initial hype analysis described is, perhaps, just a bit unfair. Presumably, some of the articles describe truly innovative contributions to deep medicine. In such cases, it would be appropriate for those abstracts to have higher rates of promotional language. So, another approach to evaluating hype might be to see if the proportion of promotional sentences correlates with the best reported AUC score in the abstract. To test this theory, I took a random sample of 100 abstracts and made the comparison. Two were excluded for being irrelevant, and the remaining composed the Random-98 data set. As it turns out, there is no significant association between the percentage of promotional sentences and the best AUC score.[39] While this is not great news for the state of hype in health AI, it offers another way to account for the distribution of hype overall. Figure 5.2 compares abstracts by the percentage of promotional sentences and the highest reported AUC. Using the same genre threshold, we can say that abstracts with fewer than 20% promotional sentences are at low risk of being hype. However, the moderate risk category shifts to only those abstracts where the promotional percentage is between 20% and 40% and the AUC is over 0.9 or outstanding. Thus, the high-risk category becomes any abstract with greater than 20% promotional sentences where AUC < 0.9 or any abstract greater than 40% promotional. Within Random-98, 36.7% were classified as low risk, 29.6% as moderate risk, and 23.5% as high risk. The remaining 10.2% were unclassifiable as no specific AUC scores were reported.

Figure 5.2 also identifies which abstracts reported an external validation exercise. The quality of a study cannot, of course, be reduced to its AUC score. Unfortunately, external validation is both relatively rare and evenly distributed throughout the data set. It does not reliably account for higher rates of promotional language. Additionally, using Random-98, I evaluated the abstracts for descriptions of groundtruthing approaches: 52% were dredged, 31.6% were engineered, and 1.02% were forged. The remaining abstracts (15.3%) did not report enough information about groundtruthing

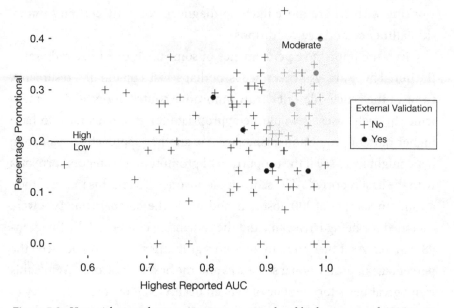

Figure 5.2. Hype risk zones by percentage promotional and highest reported AUC.

to identify the approach. Generally, the abstracts that did not discuss groundtruthing details focused primarily on model architecture, multi-model comparisons, ensembling approaches, and tuning parameters. An evaluation of the relative percentage of promotional sentences by approach to ground truth showed that there was no meaningful difference, except in the case of forged ground truth. However, since there was only one example of forged ground truth in the data set, no conclusions can be drawn from these data. See Figure 5.3.

However, there were many examples of forged ground truth in the Training Set used for HypeDx. The 82 articles were 7.32% dredged, 53.7% engineered, and 39.0% forged. Based on the percentage of promotional language and the highest reported AUC scores, 43.18% of engineered articles and 68.75% of forged articles were in the zone for high risk of hype. This difference is statistically significant.[40] At the same time, the average max AUC of forged articles was notably higher than those for engineered articles with a mean difference of 0.0632.[41] See Figure 5.4 for more details. So forged articles were both more likely to return a higher AUC and more likely to be in the high-risk

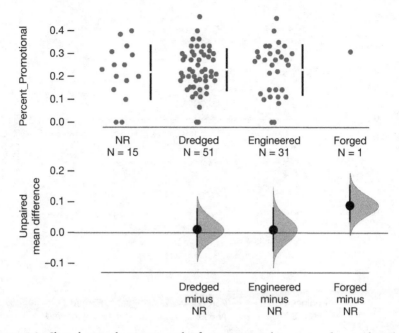

Figure 5.3. Shared control estimation plot for promotional percent and ground truth approach.

zone, making them especially dangerous. This follows from concerns in the last chapter about the bearing capacity limitations of forged ground truth. It's simply much easier to effect the appearance of a solid foundation for model training when the ground truth is forged rather than dredged or engineered. The good news is that forged groundtruthing does not appear to be all that common in the random sample of articles. However, it is overrepresented in Lieu et al.'s meta-study. If meta-studies evaluating the overall performance of AI in health are built significantly on analysis of articles that lack firm bearing capacity, then this raises concerns for the quality of health AI meta-discourse.

HEDGEDX

One thing that the current hype analysis leaves out is the possibility of mitigating language. Linguists and informal logicians have devoted

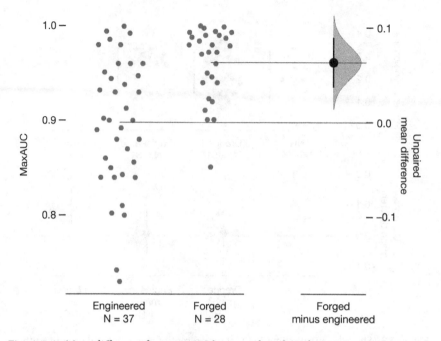

Figure 5.4. Mean difference for max AUC by ground truth in the training set.

considerable time and energy to theorizing the qualifier or the hedge. Modal verbs and qualifying adjectives and adverbs blunt the force of a claim, at least in theory. That is, "the new AI system will revolutionize clinical care" is a stronger claim than "the new AI system could possibly revolutionize clinical care." The modal verb (could) and the qualifying adverb (possibly) do much to reduce the strength of the claim and therefore, potentially, limit the extent to which one of the latter sentences might qualify as hype. There is, however, a problem with this analysis. Empirical research into the audience reception of hedges in scientific claims tends to show that hedging causes audiences to confer credibility.[42] The braggart scientist is less trustworthy than the one who carefully hedges claims. Given this, hedging actually confers additional risks to hype. If hype is moderated with credibility markers in the form of hedges, then it is possible that hyped research could be seen as very trustworthy.

When we see a measured account of extravagant claims, we start to question if what we are reading is, indeed, hype. This is a feature, not a bug. Effective hype relies on careful hedging to disrupt the notion that you are being sold a bill of goods.[43] An overt advertising pitch is seldom successful because as soon as you feel yourself being persuaded, psychological reactance kicks in.[44] You mentally resist. Consider the trope of the used car sales professional: "Zero to 60 in 4 seconds! 100 miles to the gallon! Will secure your chosen partner! Only \$12,999!" If you are like me, "LEMON ALERT!" is flashing in your mind. Psychological reactance is also why reverse psychology often works in young children. "You can't tell me what to do!" is a classic movement of reactance. As mentioned above, the social scientific literature shows that hedging can decrease reactance and increase trust. Thus, the primary effect of the hedging while hyping is performative. You cannot dub AI more important than railroads without raising a few eyebrows. A few carefully leveraged hedges tend to make an argument appear more reasonable and the audience more open to persuasion.

In order to explore this issue further, I trained another binary classifier to identify hedging in abstracts from articles about health AI. The same team of raters used the same training set to annotate hedged claims about AI systems. The interrater reliability was 94% agreement, $\kappa = .673$ or substantial agreement. I also reconciled these disagreements and used a similar bagged CART model to train the HedgeDx classifier. The final accuracy was AUC = .08012.[45] Given the more modest bearing capacity of the interrater reliability, the true performance of HedgeDx is likely below AUC = 0.8. The big risk with hedged language is that it correlates with promotional language. If hedging increases alongside hype, it suggests that the hedge is a credibility move and not claim strength moderation. Unfortunately, this is exactly what we see in the PubMed-973 data set. That is, when hedging is present, the rates increase in tandem hype rates.[46] Fortunately, however, few of the articles in the data set include hedging, so there is not a large cause for concern in this respect. Nevertheless, it is important to be mindful that hedging can function as something as a hype get-out-of-jail-free card, and that is precisely why it cannot be treated as such.

CONCLUSION

Ultimately, the findings presented here suggest that while hype is a common feature in health AI, it is not hugely dominant. In the performance-correcting analysis of the Random-100 data set, nearly a quarter of articles were at high risk of hype. This is a substantial proportion, but it still leaves the bulk of the available research at moderate or low risk. Perhaps more importantly, the findings here indicate that it is possible to identify hype based on a few salient features. HypeDx can determine the distribution of promotional sentences in abstracts. When these data are combined with performance metrics and methodological details, separating out the hyped research may not be so difficult. In so doing, readers of health AI should be on the lookout for articles that lack external validation and that rely on forged ground truth (especially if forged through a problematic consensus-based approach). Additionally, readers of research on health AI should be on the lookout for hedges that may lend credibility to overhyped research findings. Academic training often focuses attention on methodological features and statistical literacy when it comes to teaching early career researchers to interpret abstracts. Additionally, training early career researchers to look out for potentially problematic rhetorical features may improve both overall technical literacy and peer review practices.

Beyond individual articles, however, the results presented in this chapter indicate that there may be bigger problems with hype in the aggregate. That is, broad-based discussions about AI that are not grounded in specific studies of specific technologies may be more likely to overstate the benefits of AI. Liu et al.'s meta-analysis ultimately finds "diagnostic performance of deep learning models to be equivalent to that of health-care professionals."[47] But this finding is based on a data set that overrepresents the distribution of potentially problematic approaches to ground truth. Certain consensus-based approaches to forged ground truth can substantially overestimate the bearing capacity of that ground truth and lead to hyperbolic claims about system performance and to correspondingly misplaced surety in oracular AI. Fortunately, the oracular rubric is not the only rubric. Some advocates of deep medicine are also actively pursuing technologies designed to address more systemic issues. Certainly, these are not without their own problems. Tech fixes for inequity raise serious justice and ethical concerns. Yet perhaps, in some cases, justice-oriented systems may be warranted as a temporary solution. These are the issues I will address in the next chapter.

Ethics, Justice, and Health AI

On a scale of 1–10, how much pain do you feel right now?

This simple question, which is asked millions of times a day throughout the world, is the state of the art in pain measurement. The Numeric Pain Rating Scale (NPRS) and its cousin, the Visual Analog Scale (VAS)— sketches of progressively sadder smiley faces—are the primary ways that doctors assess pain. NPRS and VAS are low-tech quantitization regimes that assist with the practice of pain management. Just like my introductory example of Matthew McConaughey's versus my attractiveness, the NPRS and the VAS assign a number to sensory experience. They do not *measure* that experience in any meaningful sense of the word. Importantly, the NPRS and the VAS were not designed to quantify a moment in pain. They were designed to guide treatment. If your shoulder used to hurt a level 6, but daily stretching makes it hurt at level 3, we know that physical therapy is working.

Despite the fact that the NPRS and VAS scales are the gold standard approach to pain management, the inability to measure pain directly is a regular lament of clinicians in many areas of medicine. During interviews I conducted as part of a previous study of pain medicine, the desire for pain measurement or "algometry" was a recurrent theme. One interventional anesthesiology informant expressed frustration that he didn't "have a way of hooking someone up to a pain-o-meter. We can measure pain behavior, but pain behavior is obviously very personalized."[1] Likewise, an

The Doctor and the Algorithm. S. Scott Graham, Oxford University Press. © Oxford University Press 2022.
DOI: 10.1093/oso/9780197644461.003.0007

orthopedist suggested that "one of the first things those concerned will admit [is] there's no algometer, no dial on somebody's forehead. As long as you can't read it out, you have to rely on the patient's report."[2] Importantly, these are remarks from pain management specialists with long-standing investments in what is known as the "biopsychosocial" model of pain.[3] That is, their daily clinical practices are marked by a commitment to the idea that pain lives at the intersection of biological, psychological, and social processes. They would be among the first to reject the idea that pain should be understood as merely physical. And yet, the desire for an "objective" measurement that escapes the limitations of patient self-report remains. This desire for objectivity, combined with the common denigration of patient report as "merely subjective," unfortunately, creates a situation where systemic marginalization and implicit biases often run amok in pain medicine.

Increasingly, AI is being offered as a possible intervention for such systemic inequities. In the context of pain management specifically, recent studies have offered what they hope will be that missing "dial on the forehead." This chapter is devoted to exploring these two interventions. Specifically, I will address one AI system designed to measure pain in noncommunicating patients[4] and a second that offers to "correct" implicit racial biases in clinical care.[5] The idea that one can use AI to intervene in ongoing inequities has been around for a while. However, as previous chapters have shown, the rush to act amid technochauvinist logics can lead to ill-considered and dangerous systems that perpetuate the issues the architects sought to redress. Knowing when to build, when not to build, and how to develop proposed solutions to systemic problems ethically is critical if AI wishes to work toward more fair or just clinical worlds. Much has been written in critical algorithm studies that can help guide the way. However, since so little of that work directly addresses clinical contexts, it is essential that ethical recommendations be appropriately attenuated to the particularities of clinical medicine. So, in what follows, I begin by outlining the most prominent approaches to better AI and then explore what the aforementioned case studies in AI algometry suggest for the development of ethical approaches to deep medicine.

TOWARD BETTER AI

AI has been shown time and time again to be a remarkable engine for codifying and accelerating structural inequalities. The examples of WMDs in the Introduction to this book or in the collected literature of critical algorithm studies should be enough to make anyone recognize the need for change. We are at a moment that quite simply requires a "moral imagination . . . to explicitly embed better values into our algorithms, creating Big Data models that follow our ethical lead."[6] And there is at least some good news on this front. As we are becoming increasingly aware of the many dangers of AI, there has been a proliferation of initiatives in industry, nonprofit sectors, academia, and occasionally government—all devoted to better AI. We cannot really say that we are short on moral imagination at this point. In fact, I would go so far as to say that we are vexed by a dizzying array of competing moral imaginations. Ethics and justice-based frameworks for AI's moral future vie for attention in industry, academic, and media landscapes, leaving technologists with an expansive menu of options. But like the items on any menu, not all are of equal nutritive (moral) value. There's good reason to believe that much of Ethical AI in industry and some academic spaces is little more than window dressing.[7] It's hand-waving at a vision of fairness that's ultimately subordinated to innovation and profit. There's also good reason to think that some of the recommendations of Just AI may not be fully appropriate for clinical contexts.[8]

In this chapter, I will think about the various approaches to better AI as existing along two intersecting spectra: an ethical-just spectrum and a governance-intervention spectrum. These two spectra intersect to create a sort of coordinate system that can serve usefully (if incompletely) to map the many versions of better AI. As I describe how different approaches to better AI fit on these intersecting spectra, I will be focusing on two wings of the first spectrum: Ethical AI and Just AI. Each of these wings has both governance-focused and interventional-focused initiatives. To speak in broad strokes, Ethical AI governance is generally focused on transparency and audibility. That is, adherents of Ethical AI recommend structures and

Table 6.1. GOVERNANCE AND INTERVENTIONAL FOCI FOR
ETHICAL AND JUST AI

	Governance	Interventional AI
Ethical AI	Transparency, interpretability, auditability, self-governance	Algorithmic fairness, diverse training sets
Just AI	Precaution, regulation	Abolitionist tools, counter-data

mechanisms that make it possible to identify and understand the harms of new technologies. Interventional Ethical AI tends to focus on technical solutions like algorithmic fairness and diverse training data. In contrast, Just AI centers on precaution and emancipation. More specifically, Just AI governance tends to suggest that unless a new technology is explicitly emancipatory (antiracist, anti-sexist, anti-ableist, etc.), then serious, protracted, and community-engaged considerations of the potential harms must precede development. Table 6.1 outlines my way of thinking about some of the key foci for each of the quadrants created by these intersecting spectra as they are embodied by the Ethical and Just wings. In what follows, I outline some of these distinctions in a bit more detail.

As mentioned previously, on the extreme ethical end of the Ethical AI spectrum, we tend to see a strong focus on transparency and auditability. This version of Ethical AI imagines a world where companies of the tech industry have a fiduciary and perhaps also legal responsibility to evaluate and mitigate against the potential harms of new products. O'Neil outlines this model directly in *Weapons of Math Destruction*:

Generally speaking, the job of algorithmic accountability should start with the companies that develop algorithms. They should accept responsibility for their influence and develop evidence that what they're doing isn't causing harm, just as chemical companies need to provide evidence that they are not destroying the rivers and watersheds around them. That's not to say that algorithms should be universally outlawed or forced open source, but it does mean that the burden of proof rests on companies, which should be required to audit their algorithms for legality, fairness, and accuracy.[9]

Notably, the primary locus of ethical activity is within the company. It is the responsibility of corporations to ensure that their tech is ethical. They may be called upon by external regulators to provide "proof" of non-harm, but again they are the curators and caretakers of that proof.

Within this version of Ethical AI, a significant focus is the tech audit. Such accountability exercises would focus on asking key questions about the potential harms of new products. Glossing Data & Society's primer of algorithmic accountability, Benjamin articulates three essential questions for any AI audit: "What are the unintended consequences of designing systems at scale on the basis of existing patterns in society? When and how should AI systems prioritize individuals over society and vice versa? When is introducing an AI system the right answer—and when is it not?"[10] Raji, Smart, et al. offer a particularly promising "end-to-end" framework for internal audits from an Ethical AI perspective.[11] The proposed audit schema includes some of the best recommendations of Just AI, especially in terms of center stakeholder involvement and social impact assessments. One core difference between this framework and the recommendations of Just AI is the timing of stakeholder involvement. Community inclusion is a critical first step of the audit, but the audit comes after investments in product development. The schema assumes that product design will produce auditable artifacts that a stakeholder and social impacts–focused assessment can evaluate.

In addition to the question of when to center auditing activities, the question of who should conduct these audits helps to define the continuum between Ethical and Just approaches. Locating ethical divisions within tech companies is, quite obviously, a double-edged sword. Certainly, companies in the tech business are in the best position to discern whether their products will be harmful prior to development and/or launch. Yet, trusting these companies to prioritize fairness over profit, as O'Neil recommends, seems like a lot to expect. In contrast, Benjamin argues that "audits need to be independent and enforceable," thus hinting at a regulatory approach.[12] The aforementioned Data & Society primer outlines roles for journalists, academics, whistleblowers, and regulators alike.[13] Just approaches to AI, on the other hand, tend to shift from transparency and

auditability (which imply products complete or in development) to a precautionary model for the tech industry. In Thomas Mullaney's introduction to *Your Computer Is on Fire*, he notes that "Fire also signals a state of
crisis. Whether in the context of criminal justice, accelerating ecological
crisis, access to credit and capital, governance, or elsewhere, computation
and new media increasingly have life-or-death consequences."[14] AI is an
emergency. People are being hurt and killed right now. As a result, we
have a moral responsibility to stop and take stock of what AI is doing and
where AI is headed. Kvita Philip argues in the closing chapter of the same
volume that we simply have to slow down. As she writes, "Moving fast
and breaking things works if we have enough privilege and safety not to
be affected by the loss of the things we break, and enough certainty in our
goals that we do not have to stop and worry whether we are going in the
right direction."[15]

Importantly, the fire for Mullaney and his co-editors and coauthors is
real. It is the fire of the material impacts of long-standing inequity, and
it is also the fire of climate change, that reinforces and accelerates those
inequities. The world is burning in no small part due to the climactic
impacts of media technologies and AI. While precautionary approaches
to AI have been a part of Just AI discourse for some time, in tying AI
to environmental justice, there is increased resonance with the precautionary principle. In short, the precautionary principle suggests that new
technologies should not be developed or introduced as long as the potential harms are unknown. This principle is a frequent feature of environ-
mentalist and environmental justice discourse, especially in the contexts
of genetically modified organizations and climate change. With respect to
AI, the precautionary principle is probably explicitly invoked most frequently with reference to lethal AI—war and police robots.[16] Whether explicit or not, a focus on precaution is apparent in other areas of Just AI
discourse. For example, when we celebrate IBM for ending facial recognition software development[17] or Microsoft for refusing to sell facial recognition technology to the police,[18] then we are celebrating a precautionary
approach.

Perhaps nowhere is the environmentally based precautionary approach more readily apparent than in Bender, Gebru, McMillan-Major, and Mitchells' "On the Dangers of Stochastic Parrots: Can Language Models Be Too Big?"[19] Training large language models is expensive—economically, computationally, and environmentally. The computing industry is responsible for a full 2% of global carbon emissions.[20] And the supercomputers that are used to train AI and large language models like BERT are prolific emitters. Recent estimates place the total carbon output of supercomputers in Australia at 15 kilotons for astronomy alone.[21] Given this kind of output, Bender et al. raise serious questions about how to factor environmental injustice into the development of large language models:

> On the one hand, it is well documented in the literature on environmental racism that the negative effects of climate change are reaching and impacting the world's most marginalized communities first [1, 27]. Is it fair or just to ask, for example, that the residents of the Maldives (likely to be underwater by 2100 [6]) or the 800,000 people in Sudan affected by drastic floods [7] pay the environmental price of training and deploying ever larger English LMs, when similar large-scale models aren't being produced for Dhivehi or Sudanese Arabic?[22]

Ultimately, the authors argue for a precautionary approach. While they do not explicitly invoke the precautionary principle, they make a clear claim for "a reallocation of efforts towards approaches that avoid some of these risks while still reaping the benefits of improvements to language technology."[23]

Just and Ethical AI offer a wide range of potential frameworks, and there is great potential to bring these frameworks to bear productively on deep medicine. However, prominent works in critical algorithm studies offer scant attention to AI in health and medicine. Neither "health" nor "medicine" make the indexes of *Artificial Unintelligence*, *Algorithms of Oppression*, or *Your Computer Is on Fire*. This is not a critique of any of these books or authors.[24] The other sectors they chose to address demanded and continue to demand our attention. Nevertheless, the relative lack of attention to health AI makes it hard to argue with those who suggest that the ethical recommendations of algorithmic fairness are not well attenuated to medicine.[25] As just one example, Alex John London also points out that the rush to fold Ethical or Just AI into clinical contexts may result in unintended patient harm.[26] Specifically, he notes how calls for eXplainable AI (XAI) may result in overestimating the explainability of human medical decision-making and can lead to diminished accuracy. There are a lot of things that doctors know work, but they don't know *how* they work. Randomized controlled trials are designed to provide evidence of efficacy, but not an account of mechanism of action, or as London puts it, "the ability to explain how results are produced can be less important than the ability to produce such results and empirically verify their accuracy."[27]

The simple truth is that the black boxes of medicine often perform better than more explainable systems. This includes both AI systems and pharmacological systems. When it comes to healthcare, I personally want the intervention that's most likely to make me better, even if my doctor can't quite explain how it works. Within this context, London ultimately argues that

> Recommendations to prioritize explainability or interpretability over predictive and diagnostic accuracy are unwarranted in domains where our knowledge of underlying causal systems is lacking. Such recommendations can result in harms to patients whose diseases go undiagnosed or who are exposed to unnecessary additional testing.[28]

This is, importantly, not intended as a license for a deep medicine free-for-all. London cautions that AI must be used judiciously and only in appropriate cases. Nevertheless, Ethical and Just AI's common focus on XAI does always not sit comfortably with best practices in clinical care. And, of course, there is the problem that XAI often leads to undue trust in system recommendations. See Chapter 2 of this book for more details on this issue.

Critically, this chapter is simply not going to drop a new framework into the mix that magically resolves these tensions. As Philip points out in the closing chapter to *Your Computer Is on Fire*, there are no easy answers here. When confronted by the complex reality of real-world cases, codified ethical frameworks quickly fall apart. As she notes,

> A priori rules for ethics and logical axiomatic frameworks for describing technology's operation are useful for some kinds of documentation but counterproductive in most everyday messy examples of real life. We can only get the complexity we need to navigate a crowded technological theater on fire through collaboration, conversation, and rigorous exploration of the strands of modernity's multivalent skein.[29]

The AI algometry cases I discuss next are precisely the kind of everyday messy examples that make ethical work here such a challenge. However, these are instructive cases precisely because they do not lead to easy conclusions. They showcase the limitations of current frameworks but also highlight the significant difficulties in doing this work. The current spectrum of approaches for better AI can make it difficult to select the best course of action (including the possibility of no action). In some cases, Ethical and Just frameworks end up recommending divergent approaches. An ethical and just deep medicine must be ready to confront these potential conflicts.

ABLEISM AND AI ALGOMETRY

Because this book is so indebted to critical algorithm studies and related strands of critical race theory (CRT), much of my attention to structural marginalization has focused on racism in health and medicine. But, quite obviously, race is not the only dimension of inequity in medicine or society at large. One area not yet well addressed in this book is ableism in medicine. In many respects, contemporary Western medicine is a normalizing engine. It indexes health to idealized exemplars of able-bodiedness and treats all deviations as deficits to be corrected. Subsequently, significant bodies of research have shown how ableism pervades clinical practice.[30] One of the most significant impacts of medical ableism is physician biases surrounding quality of life. That is, doctors routinely assume that patients with disabilities necessarily experience diminished quality of life because of those disabilities. This assumption can result in reduced quality of care. Tragically, ableism in medicine has been shown to cause people with disabilities to fear or avoid care. This issue was essentially prominent during the COVID-19 pandemic where there was a real concern that these clinical biases in the context of overtaxed hospitals would lead to a denial of care for people with disabilities.[31] In the contexts of pain management, ableism can lead to undertreatment, especially in situations where clinicians are not sufficiently prepared for patients with complex communication needs.[32] Effectively addressing ableism in medicine will require significant, long-term structural and educational interventions. Clinicians must be better prepared to address ethically the needs of patients with disabilities, and AI has been offered as one way to assist with these efforts.

Specifically, a 2015 study led by researchers from the University of Ulm in Germany developed an AI system designed to measure pain directly from physiological response. According to the resulting *PLOS ONE* article, the motivations for the study were two-fold. First, they aimed to create a machine that could better achieve commonly accepted scientific targets for "objective and robust measurement."[33] And, second, the authors hoped to address the pressing need of assessing patient pain among those who cannot report. The introduction remarks on clinicians' need for patients to be "sufficiently alert and cooperative" and suggests that this may not be possible for "people with verbal and/or cognitive impairments," or "people who are sedated and automated ventilated."[34] While I would be among the first to agree that clinicians absolutely need the ability to assess pain for cognitively impaired and post-surgical patients, the phraseology here is obviously concerning. "Sufficiently . . . cooperative" is a huge red flag in terms of patient agency and autonomy. However, I am going to set that aside for just a moment to describe the larger study design.

Ultimately, Gruss et al.'s study was an exercise in supervised machine learning. As discussed in previous chapters, this involves training a statistical model (in this case a support vector machine [SVM]) to discern patterns in one data set based on labels provided by the research team. Given the aim of developing reliable algometry for nonverbal patients, the data used for pattern recognition are based on physiological response. Primarily this involved measures of electrical muscle activity, skin conductance, heart rate, and heart rate variability. The labeling data for the training and testing sets was created by directly inducing pain with a specialized device that is essentially the equivalent of a rapid-acting soldering iron. Researchers outfitted each study participant with (a) a "thermal stimulator" attached to the forearm and (b) an emergency shutoff button to be used when in pain. In a series of tests, researchers cranked up the heat until each participant experienced pain and hit the button. All the while, the biopotential monitoring system collected the aforementioned data on muscle activity, skin conductance, and heart rate. In the end, the researchers were able to create a system with over 90% accuracy in distinguishing between pain and no pain. Interestingly, the high accuracy was based primarily on what sounds an awful lot like wincing. That is, when there were high degrees of signal similarity in the electrical activity for two facial muscles (the zygomaticus and corrugator), the SVM system could reliably identify a pain response.

The problematic language of patient "compliance" notwithstanding, this study seems as though it could have some real potential to help patients who are unconscious or who face other barriers preventing them from communicating their pain effectively. Pain management based on patient report is the gold standard, but it is certainly a problem when reporting is not possible. In fact, recognition of this challenge has recently prompted the International Association for the Study of Pain (IASP) to change its long-standing definition of pain. In 1979, the IASP convened the 4th World Congress on Pain to sketch out an operational definition of pain that could inform pain management in surgery, palliative care, dentistry, and all manner of clinical and research settings. The congressional delegates developed a definition grounded in multidisciplinary consensus that set the standard in pain medicine for decades. The short version of the definition is as follows: "An unpleasant sensory and emotional experience associated with actual or potential tissue damage, or described in terms of such damage."[35] Many have decried the centrality of "description" in this definition as suggesting that self-report is a necessary precondition for pain. For example, one researcher concerned with pain management for newborns argued that

> This definition requires patients to describe their pain, by default establishing the primacy of self-report as a "gold standard." Although widely accepted across all healthcare professions and biomedical disciplines, this definition lacks applicability to non-verbal populations and ignores the cognitive and social dimensions of pain.[36]

This critique has been rejected on a number of grounds, including that it misunderstands the meaning the word "or" in "or described in terms of such damage."[37] From my perspective, the most compelling objection to this criticism is that the original IASP definition included the following explanatory note: "Note: The inability to communicate verbally does not negate the possibility that an individual is experiencing pain and is in need of appropriate pain-relieving treatment."[38]

Nevertheless, the IASP revised its definition to respond to these complaints and other issues in 2020. The new definition reads as follows: "An unpleasant sensory and emotional experience associated with, or resembling that associated with, actual or potential tissue damage."[39] Alongside this definition, the IASP offers six key notes that further refine and clarify the definition. Generally, these notes focus on valorizing the complex, multifaceted, and biopsychosocial nature of pain. One note is particularly important for attempts to develop AI algometry: "Pain and nociception[40] are different phenomena. Pain cannot be inferred solely from activity in sensory neurons." While this note only specifically identifies "activity in sensory neurons" as an inappropriate foundation for pain inference, it certainly implies that physiological inference, writ large, may be problematic. If pain is fundamentally and irreducibly biopsychosocial and, as note #4 directs, "A person's report of an experience as pain should be respected," the very idea of AI algometry becomes increasingly suspect. The drive for "objective" pain measurement recenters pain in physiological processes and marginalizes the psychosocial aspects to deny patient agency and autonomy.

Ultimate, I think Gruss et al.'s system is a textbook example of Ethical AI in a clinical context. Ethical AI tends to preserve a bias toward action. The ethical vision is grounded in the presumption that companies will build things. Thus, governance solutions and interventional technologies alike are engineered to guide (rather than prevent) that action. For the most part, interventional Ethical AI focuses on technologically engineered solutions to algorithmic bias. For example, one of the canonical works of Ethical AI proposes the following definition of anti-classification in Ethical AI:

$$d(x) = d(x') \text{ for all x, x' such that } x_u = x'_u \text{ }^{41}$$

In English, "anti-classification" is largely a matter of not including identifying characteristics (including ethnic data) in AI systems. Of course, as many in critical algorithm studies have pointed out, the complex effects of systemic racism can create surrogate data points for race, such as zip code, that blunt a narrower approach to anti-classification. Much like the case with Ethical AI governance, interventional fairness solutions tend to be in-house. In recent years, IBM, Facebook, and Google have all deployed new computational libraries designed to detect bias or engineer fairness in their algorithms.[42] Technologically oriented solutionism is precisely what allows some areas of Ethical AI to offer an apparently ethical intervention that is still ultimately subordinated to the dominant market logics of the corporation.

In much the same way, Gruss et al.'s system is an act of Ethical AI. To be sure, it is not situated in a corporate context, but it ultimately offers a tech fix that subordinates emancipatory aims to dominant clinical logics. When confronted with the problem of noncommunicating patients, the system architects look for a way to short-circuit the troubling need for patient report and thus recenter pain on physiological responses to nociception. Developing effective methods for inferring pain in nonverbal patients is a critical ethical demand, and this system (although quite problematic) may end up offering some help to some patients. Yet at the same time, centering pain in traditional domains of biomedical expertise (the body) is a troubling intervention in a clinical area that has been marked by long-standing physician distrust of already marginalized people. This is all the more troubling when understood through a rubric of "compliance." When "objective" algometry recenters "true" pain in the domain of the physician, it becomes even easier to weaponize so-called "noncompliance."

RACISM AND AI ALGOMETRY

Of course, racism continues to be a significant and enduring problem in American medicine, and pain management is no exception. As mentioned in the Introduction, a 2016 survey of medical trainees found that 73% believed at least one false statement about race-based biological differences.[43] Among the most striking statistics was the fact that 58% believed that Black skin is thicker than white skin. This false belief and others like it have been traced directly to inequalities in pain management. Physicians routinely underestimate patient pain across patient groups, but the racial differences are striking. Doctors are twice as likely to underestimate Black pain.[44] As a result, Black patients are less likely to receive pain medication, and when they do, they routinely receive lower quantities than white patients.[45] As these disparities are increasingly recognized by the medical community, recommendations for improvement tend to center around a mix of implicit bias training and increased reliance on more "objective" diagnostic technologies. The American Association of Medical Colleges, for example, recommends that in addition to implicit bias training, clinical guidelines should "remove as much individual discretion as possible," and researchers should "continue the search for objective measures of pain."[46]

The architects of a new algometry AI have developed a system they hope will both provide more objective pain measures and lead to reduced clinical biases.[47] Working with a diverse population of osteoarthritis of the knee patients, the researchers "trained a convolutional neural network to predict the reported pain score for each knee using each X-ray image, using a randomly selected training and development data set of 25,049 radiographs (2,877 patients)."[48] The developed algorithmic pain prediction (ALG-P) system identifies key features in collected X-rays and interprets those features based on training labels from patient pain reports. The study team compared ALG-P estimates of pain severity with those of the preexisting industry standard clinical decision tool, Kellgren–Lawrence Grade (KLG). The KLG, which was developed and validated on a predominantly white British population in 1957, guides human evaluation of X-rays for osteoarthritis of the knee.[49] ALG-P was 61% more accurate in estimating patient pain than the KLG. Importantly, however, while the ALG-P reduces the frequency and magnitude of racial disparities, it does not eliminate them. So, if a Black patient had a true pain level of 8, a doctor using KLG might estimate the pain at level 6, and one using the ALG-P might estimate it at a 7.

The ALG-P and the design of this study live up to some of the best-practice recommendations for Just AI. One common recommendation for a more just approach to AI is to ensure that training data is labeled by members of the communities who will be most affected by the system and its use. Community-provided labeling data is one partial solution to the problem of privilege hazard discussed in Chapter 1. A pervasive problem in pain medicine is that physicians tend to believe their own estimates of patient pain over those from patient report. By training ALG-P on labeling data from patient report, the developers artfully sidestep this issue. In an interview with the MIT Technology Review, one of the study authors, Ziad Obermeyer, highlighted this more just approach as central to the study:

"That was exactly the secret," agrees Obermeyer. If algorithms are only ever trained to match expert performance, he says, they will simply perpetuate existing gaps and inequities. "This study is a glimpse of a more general pipeline that we are increasingly able to use in medicine for generating new knowledge."[50]

Ultimately, both the study itself and some of the related media coverage indicate a hope that the availability of these data might encourage self-reflection, leading to reduced clinical biases. As the study points out, "cooperation between humans and algorithms was shown to improve clinical decision making in some settings."[51] The previously mentioned *MIT Technology Review* article is even more enthusiastic, suggesting that "AI could make health care fairer—by helping us believe what patients say."[52] However, living up to one principle of Just AI does not necessarily assure that a given AI leads to justice.

As a scholar with long-standing interests in pain medicine, I am getting a powerful sense of déjà vu here. Doctors suddenly "trusting" patients when a shiny new technology comes along and "proves" those patients right is becoming an all-too-familiar narrative. Almost 20 years ago, the case du jour was fibromyalgia—a chronic widespread bodily pain condition believed to be caused by an inability to regulate properly certain nerve signals. Fibromyalgia disproportionately afflicts women, another group many doctors seem to have trouble believing. A 2003 *Newsweek* article effectively captures the narrative similarities here:

Until recently, doctors didn't believe fibromyalgia pain was real. They thought it was "all in the heads" of sufferers, who happened to be mainly women. When Dr. Muhammad Yunus of the University of Illinois began studying it in 1977, colleagues warned him, "You'll ruin your career. These women are just crazy." But the fact that doctors couldn't find a cause or a cure for some 6 million sufferers didn't mean that the pain wasn't there. In the past few years scientists have used powerful brain scans to provide proof that it is.[53]

Then-recent advances in neuroimaging technologies, specifically positron emission tomography (PET), were able to identify differences in how some people's brains process certain stimuli. With an "objective" technologically enabled finding now available, "trust" in patient report became possible.

Now, for many, this version of "trust" does not sound a whole lot like genuine trust. If trust is only granted when verified through technological "objectivity," then there is no trust at all. What's more, the average cost of a PET scan in 2020 is just over $5,000.[54] Even if insurance is reimbursing these costs, that is a pretty steep fee for "trusting" women. Similarly, it is not clear how much money it cost to develop ALG-P, but some combination of direct funding and salary support was provided by the Social Security Administration, the Department of Defense, and Microsoft Research. Specific dollar values aside, this seems like an awful lot of time, energy, and money for a product that offers a 61% accuracy improvement when believing Black patients would offer a 100% accuracy improvement.

Obviously, I am being quite critical in my analysis here, and that's not exactly where I want to end this chapter. Reflecting on these two cases in AI algometry, I am struck by several contradictory facts:

1. Physicians need better resources for assessing pain in nonverbal patients.
2. Technologies that infer pain from physiological processes risk valorizing expert assessment over patient report.
3. Right at this moment, patients are receiving inadequate treatment for pain due to systematic racism, ableism, and associated implicit biases.
4. Technologically validated trust is not trust at all.

Amid these conflicting yet true statements, I find it genuinely difficult to settle on a final evaluation of AI algometry. There are so many things wrong with contemporary medicine, and so many people in need of immediately improved medical care. These interventions are Band Aids on bullet holes. They cannot be allowed to be the end of the line in improving pain medicine. Yet, if their deployment helps improve the health of an underserved patient right now, is it ethical to reject these technologies outright?

TOWARD BETTER HEALTH AI

As mentioned above, critical algorithm studies, by and large, have focused on social media, search engines, predictive policing, credit scoring, surveillance technologies, employment screening, and the like. The most prominent exception to this critique is probably the work of Ruha Benjamin. She has a rich research agenda in justice-based approaches to bioethics;[55] however, attention to health and medicine remains somewhat limited in her *Race after Technology* and tends to focus on non-AI technologies such as the spirometer. At the time of this writing, one of the most direct moments of ethical engagement between critical algorithm studies and health AI is a short essay Benjamin published in *Science* critiquing unethical and ill-considered approaches to racial labeling data in population health.[56] The perspective offers critically important commentary on the tendency to treat race inappropriately as an isolable biological variable. Specifically, the study she critiques uses historic costs of care to predict the health needs of patients by race. In so doing, it elides the fact that Black patients receive less care and less costly care despite often having greater health needs.

Interestingly, one of the most strident critiques of the applicability of Ethical or Just AI to health AI is built on closely related arguments about the complex structural conditions of race and gender. Specifically, McCradden, Joshi, Mazawi, and Anderson point to the potential ethical limitations of algorithmic fairness in terms of health AI. This essay is a continuation of the aforementioned conversation. It specifically invokes both Benjamin's perspective in *Science* and the original article it critiques. As they note, "Solutions of algorithmic fairness have been developed to create neutral models: models designed to produce non-discriminatory predictions by constraining bias with respect to predicted outcomes for protected identities, such as race or gender."[57] Discriminatory algorithms that use race or race-proxy data (names, zip codes) have been shown to result in considerable harm in credit scoring, predictive policing, and automated employment decisions. Thus, in these cases either declining to use algorithmic technology or, at the very least, developing systems that expressly disregard race and race-proxy data is essential. However, as McCradden et al. argue, there can be adverse health outcomes associated with such moves in healthcare contexts. As they note, "biological differences between genders can affect the efficacy of pharmacological compounds; incorporating these differences into prescribing practices does not make those prescriptions unjust."[58]

Ultimately a primary argument of this chapter is that Ethical AI and Just AI need to come together in conversation. Each area of inquiry has critically important insights that can contribute to navigating the messy complexity of messy reality. Clinical bioethics is always walking a fine line between what is best for the patient right now and for public health. Indeed, an entire 13-page chapter of the American Medical Association's (AMA) *Code of Medical Ethics* is devoted to addressing potential ethical conflicts between individual patients and society.[59] Along the way, the AMA is quick to tackle directly the potential discord between privacy obligations or patient autonomy and protecting public health. The COVID-19 pandemic brings these issues into sharp relief as doctors, epidemiologists, and politicians debate the merits and drawbacks of immunity passports and mandatory vaccination. Unfortunately, the AMA's guidance on health disparities fails to offer any clear approach to weighing potentially contradictory obligations. Rather, it provides simple directives like "avoid stereotyping patients," and "encourage shared decision making."[60] Bioethics' primary location in clinical medicine means that it has a strong commitment to methodological individualism[61] that can manifest in structural impediments to pursuing social justice.[62] Where critical algorithm studies' lack of attention to health and medicine needs to be buttressed by bioethics, bioethics could use additional insights with respect to how to address social justice on structural levels.

Deep medicine requires a careful, thoughtful, and interdisciplinary ethical formulation that attenuates the recommendations of Ethical and Just

AI to the particular needs of clinical care. The tech fix of "fair" algorithms will not be enough, but neither will broad ethical mandates developed in other technological contexts. Efforts to assure ethical and just deep medicine must proceed in concert with preexisting bioethical frameworks that are already expressly designed to address clinical contexts. In moving in this direction, McCradden, Joshi, Mazawi, and Anderson argue offer a six-point list of recommendations for "ethical approaches to issues of bias in health models of machine learning." These include:

1. Relying on neutral algorithms is problematic.
2. Problem formulation can support improved models.
3. Transparency is required surrounding model development and statistical validation.
4. Initiating transparency at point-of-care.
5. Transparency at the prediction level.
6. Ethical decision making suggests engaging diverse knowledge sources.[63]

Ultimately, these recommendations combine insights from Ethical AI, Just AI, and bioethics into an integrated framework. Here, recommendation #1 addresses the unique contexts of medicine that may require different approaches than other technology sectors in order to avoid harm. Additionally, the clarifying notes to recommendations #2, #3, and #5 invoke the common tenets of Ethical AI and point toward the importance of auditability in deep medicine. Recommendation #4 folds in long-standing bioethical commitments to the importance of informed consent/refusal, and #6 hearkens to Just AI with a focus on community-engaged tech development. In sum, these recommendations are a more thorough blending of Ethical AI and bioethics, with Just AI as a more distant partner (again, the spectrum). Ultimately, the entire framework is justified on the canonical bioethical principle of non-maleficence, i.e., the bioethical duty to do no harm, either through action or inaction. The twin sides of non-maleficence are critical to appreciating the necessity of an integrated bioethical–Just AI framework. The precautionary principle as applied in critical algorithm studies typically assumes that inaction is likely to cause the least harm. However, when structural racism and implicit biases are actively causing harm to patients right now, a partial intervention may be more morally preferable to no intervention at all. Non-maleficence is also implied by London's concerns about accuracy versus explainability. If a doctor has to choose between a more accurate intervention and a more explainable intervention, non-maleficence likely suggests she should choose the more accurate one.

While this ongoing conversation makes important strides in bringing critical algorithm studies together with bioethics and health AI, it is also clear that additional work is required in this area. This is going to have to be a sustained team effort. There are many ways to advance this conversation, and we will need to pursue all of them as a collation of communities— academic and civic. At the end of an already long chapter, I cannot address too many of these potential pathways. However, one place where I'd like to offer a modest suggestion is in the area of precaution. The doctrine of non-maleficence has the real potential to create contradictory moral inclinations when it is genuinely not clear whether action or inaction is the better course. Certainly, much of Just AI asserts a straightforward precautionary stance and is right to do so. We do not need algorithmic credit scoring. Digitally accelerating redlining offers no potential benefits, unless you consider rank profiteering a benefit. A hardline Just AI stance against algorithmic credit scoring is ethically warranted because the risk of harm clearly outweighs any possible benefit. In contrast, Black and disabled patients at the doctor need better care right now. I don't know that AI algometry necessarily provides that better care, but some advances in AI might even if they are not (yet?) Just AI. Healthcare is often defined by the best of bad options. At the same time, the recommendations of health AI and even bioethically informed health AI often simply assume that technological development will or must happen. Thus, I think an important step in bringing bioethics and Just AI together is to develop frameworks that might guide precautionary decision-making.

The conflicts created by non-maleficence in the context of uncertainty are familiar territory for bioethics. One framework for addressing these

conflicts is clinical equipoise.[64] Clinical equipoise justifies cautious exploration of new interventions in the face of genuine uncertainty between
options. Critically, it does not authorize immediate distribution to the general population. It is the moral framework upon which clinical trials—
rigorous testing of alternatives—are built. Clinical equipoise blended with
a precautionary sensibility provided by Just AI can provide a more solid
foundation for decision-making about when and if to act. Subsequently,
I close this chapter by offering my suggestion for a clinical equipoise–
inspired precautionary heuristic for deep medicine. Specifically, those
who wish to offer technological solutions to health inequity should, at the
very least, address the following questions.

- Is the proposed intervention likely to substantially address an
  unmet or under-met community need?
- Have members of the communities most likely to be affected
  by the intervention been substantively involved in project
  conceptualization, putative benefits, risk assessment, data
  curation, and training set labeling?
- Does the project team have a robust plan for evaluating
  unintended consequences during design, development, testing,
  and distribution?
- Does the project team have a robust plan for supporting long-
  term community-centered justice-oriented initiatives in this area?

If the answer is not a resounding "yes" to all of these questions, then precaution is almost certainly the way to go. However, in the context of a robust community-led approach to development, then it may be appropriate
to work at developing temporary technological fixes. That last question,
however, is key. One of the biggest risks of the tech fix is that it will be understood as a "fix." The long-term community-led work of social justice
has to continue while Band-Aid technologies offer partial improvements
in care for patients right now. Importantly, this is an internal heuristic. It
is presented as a set of questions that health technologists must address
before proceeding. But like most in Just AI, I believe ethical foundations

cannot be left solely to technologists. Regulatory oversight will always be a critical component of assuring that health innovations are safe, effective, and responsive to broad community needs. This is the major work of the next chapter. There, I will explore the most common recommendations for AI governance and regulation, the particular needs of clinical contexts, and the latest efforts of the FDA to address deep medicine.

Regulating Health AI

To date, self- and co-regulatory approaches informed by current laws and perspectives from companies, academia, and associated technical bodies have been largely successful at curbing inopportune AI use. We believe in the vast majority of instances such approaches will continue to suffice, within the constraints provided by existing governance mechanisms (e.g., sector-specific regulatory bodies).

—GOOGLE, *Perspectives on Issues in AI Governance*[1]

When I first imagined this chapter, I thought I might begin by rattling off the ever-growing litany of instances where unregulated AI has caused significant harms. I have done so several times already in this book, and in so doing I build on the careful documentary work of Benjamin, Noble, Broussard, O'Neil, Mullaney, Hicks, Philip, and many others. At this point, it is simply not hard to find evidence of harm that resulted directly from the release of ill-considered and/or unregulated AI. The ready availability of this evidence makes it all the more appalling that Google's white paper on AI governance (excerpted above) would so brazenly declare that current regulatory approaches "have been largely successful at curbing inopportune AI use." The larger document from which this passage comes is a naked attempt to blunt the potential effects of proposed AI governance

The Doctor and the Algorithm. S. Scott Graham, Oxford University Press. © Oxford University Press 2022.
DOI: 10.1093/oso/9780197644461.003.0008

and regulation. Google argues aggressively for a strong emphasis on corporate self-governance, Balkanized sector-specific regulatory bodies, and
low ceilings for damages won from successful liability litigation. The most
charitable possible read of Google's claim that current approaches have
been largely successful is that they are simply not paying attention to the
real-world consequences of their products. From my perspective, a possible lack of attention in the face of manifest harm is, by itself, more than
enough justification for a strong regulatory framework for AI. Less charitable readings make an even more compelling case.

Of course, I am certainly not alone in calls for more rigorous AI regulation. In the preceding chapter, I highlighted several such calls from
the Just AI camp. And, indeed, recent years have seen a flurry of activity from scholars, nonprofit organizations, and government agencies
alike devoted to contending with the manifest need for better AI governance. Benjamin calls for "independent and enforceable" audits.[2] Noble
argues that "public policy must address the many increasing problems
that unregulated commercial search engines pose."[3] Hicks challenges us
all to "vote for regulation."[4] And, perhaps most famously, Andrew Tutt
offers a bold proposal for "an FDA for algorithms."[5] As I am preparing
to send this manuscript to press, the United Nations has just issued a
public call for "moratoriums on the sale and use of artificial intelligence
(AI) systems until adequate safeguards are put in place."[6] While I agree
that moratoria may be appropriate for many sectors, efforts to establish
just and ethical regulatory framework need not start from scratch. In
the wake of sustained scholarly and journalistic attention to these issues,
various nonprofit and governmental agencies have promulgated a spate
of reports and white papers that sketch out possible futures for effective
AI governance. Data & Society, Oxford's Centre for the Governance of
AI, the AI Now Institute, AI4People, The Ada Lovelace Institute, the
National Science Foundation, The European Commission, and countless other entities have opened conversations or advanced proposals
as part of what the AI Now Institute calls the "first wave of policy
implementation."[7]

Running in parallel, scholars and regulators invested in deep medicine have also promulgated new regulatory frameworks for addressing
the challenges of health AI. Bioethicists and clinical methodologists have
been actively promulgating new guidelines that would transform the conduct of clinical trials, ethics review processes, and regulatory scrutiny to
better account for AI.[8] Additionally, at the time of this writing, the FDA
is currently soliciting feedback on its new proposed regulatory framework for deep medicine.[9] "Running in parallel" is the key phrase. Like
much of the scholarship discussed in this book, attention to deep medicine is largely Balkanized outside of mainstream attention to AI in other
sectors. Despite the aforementioned calls for "an FDA for AI," this division
of attention is fairly consistent when it comes to AI governance as well.
Subsequently, the driving goal of this chapter is to bring these two relatively isolated conversations more closely together. There is great potential for productive cross-pollination between AI governance broadly and
health AI regulation.

Given the relative lack of preexisting regulatory structures, broad AI
governance tends to focus on first principles and articulating the core
concerns of what it means to regulate technology in a democracy. In
contrast, given the already well-established governance frameworks of
biomedical science, attention to regulation in health AI tends to focus
on where the rubber meets the road. That is, it offers concrete, actionable steps that clearly delineate ethical demands, regulatory structures,
and lines of responsibility. In bringing these two conversations closer
together, I hope to catalyze new discussions in both areas. Ultimately,
I argue (1) that the capacious vision of broad-scale AI governance can
prompt health AI to consider productively more democratic foundations
of health governance, and (2) that the detailed recommendations for
health AI governance can accelerate efforts to build new regulatory
structures for AI broadly. In what follows, I begin with a discussion of
the core values of broad AI governance and then proceed to an exploration of targeted recommendations for governance in health AI, and finally I close this chapter by exploring the potential productive synergies
between these two lines of inquiry.

RECOMMENDATIONS FOR ALGORITHMIC GOVERNANCE

As mentioned above, scholars in critical algorithm studies have broadly called for increased AI governance. "Governance," of course, means many things, hence the careful use of "self-governance" and "co-governance" in Google's white paper. Much of the relevant scholarly literature focuses on "self-governance," particular in the context of algorithmic audits (see Chapter 6). While there are a few exceptions, the most detailed proposals for external governance or regulation come from nonprofit, think tank, research center, and government white papers. For example, Oxford's Centre for the Governance of AI has promulgated a paper outlining a targeted research agenda for AI governance.[10] Importantly, here, this document is motivated by the idea that additional research is needed to establish effective governance and therefore centers on opportunities for academic inquiry. The Data & Society primer on algorithmic accountability discussed in the last chapter also points toward external governance and regulatory possibilities. However, the overarching focus is on self-governance and the fourth estate. In the U.S. context, recommendations for AI regulation often point to Tuft's aforementioned "An FDA for Algorithms," and it is not difficult to find workshop or symposium reports like the NSF-funded Fairness, Ethics, Accountability, and Transparency (FEAT) Workshop Report.[11] Some of the most detailed proposals for AI governance come out of the EU context. The Council of Europe and The Alan Turing Institute's *Artificial Intelligence, Human Rights, Democracy, and the Rule of Law*,[12] AI4People's *On Good AI Governance*,[13] and the European Commission's white paper *On Artificial Intelligence—A European Approach to Excellence and Trust*[14] all offer somewhat more detailed recommendations for appropriate regulatory structures. As I am writing this chapter, the U.S. Federal Trade Commission (FTC) has even released new guidance calling for increased "truth, fairness, and equity" in AI and promising regulatory oversite to ensure these ends.[15]

The specifics in these articles, reports, and white papers vary widely based on focal technologies, (multi)national contexts, and espoused democratic frameworks. Nevertheless, it is possible to identify a few key overarching recommendations that are central to most regulatory proposals. Broadly, these core recommendations focus on (1) developing new frameworks that are attuned to a more expansive sense of possible harms, (2) centering community and stakeholder groups in governance and regulatory decision-making, and (3) increasing regulatory scrutiny on the earliest stages of product development. In most proposals, these key recommendations are closely interrelated. Centering community groups is identified as an important part of broadening our understanding of possible harms. Similarly, a more capacious sense of possible harms necessitates regulatory interventions earlier in product development. Given the obvious risks associated with the ill-considered deployment of AI, early life cycle regulation is a key mechanism for encouraging companies to address a broader range of potential harms up front. In what follows, I explore the particularities of the recommendations in more detail to showcase how the various recommendations are interrelated.

Recommendation #1: A more capacious sense of harms

Broadly speaking, calls for increased AI regulation center around concerns about the significant uncertainty around potential unintended consequences. AI is relatively new technology, and with any new technology, it is not always possible to predict what will happen when it is released. As the Centre on Algorithmic Governance research agenda notes, "a system of competing and cooperating agents can be amplified by novel forms of AI."[16] Similarly, this uncertain risk–benefit ratio is at the center of the European Commission's white paper on AI governance: "As with any new technology, the use of AI brings both opportunities and risks. Citizens fear being left powerless in defending their rights and safety when facing the information asymmetries of algorithmic decision-making, and companies are concerned by legal uncertainty."[17] These "information asymmetries" are a serious driver of uncertainty about the consequences of AI. It is hard to predict what a black box does.[18] And if industry aims are compromised by profit motive run amok, then there are real questions about the extent to which we can trust their in-house testing regimes. However, the aforementioned FTC guidance calls on companies to "hold yourselves accountable—or be ready for the FTC to do it for you."[19]

Traditional consumer protection schemes tend to focus on potential immediate harms to end users, and thus many advocates for AI regulation consider those schemes to be insufficient to the tasks at hand. The Council of Europe and the Alan Turing Institute's joint primer argues, in no un-certain terms, that "AI systems must not be permitted to adversely impact human wellbeing or planetary health."[20] The Centre for the Governance of AI's report even points to "risk of inadvertent nuclear war" as an issue of regulatory concern with respect to AI.[21] The primary focus, however, are risks associated with malicious use of information and communication technologies, which can be threats to "cherished rights to privacy, self-expression, association, and consent, as well as to other civil liberties and social freedoms."[22] This focus parallels the concerns of Data & Society, who point out that "there are few consumer or civil rights protections that limit the types of data used to build data profiles or that require the auditing of algorithmic decision-making."[23] The recent FTC guidance is a step in the right direction here as the agency signals that it will consider "an AI model may yield results that are unfair or inequitable to legally protected groups" to be a violation of fair trade practices.[24]

Recommendation #2: Community/Stakeholder Involvement in Governance

Given the broad potential for uncertain harms, many advocates of more rigorous algorithmic governance point to the importance of including key community and stakeholder groups in governance processes. O'Neal calls attention to this essential need in *Weapons of Math Destruction*, where she argues that community participation offers a more promising approach than the technical fixes of some versions of Ethical AI. As she writes, "[I]nstead of fighting over which single metric we should use to determine the fairness of an algorithm, we should instead try to identify the stakeholders and weigh their relative harms."[25] Likewise, both The Council of Europe and the Alan Turing Institute's joint primer and The European Commission's white paper advance citizen and stakeholder inclusion as a key component of effective AI governance. The European Commission is especially clear on this need and clearly asserts that new regulatory structures "should guarantee maximum stakeholders participation."[26] Importantly, they are clear that "stakeholders" includes "consumer organisation and social partners, businesses, researchers, and civil society organisations."[27]

Proposed mechanisms for stakeholder inclusion vary widely. The aforementioned NSF-funded FEAT workshop points to community-embedded social science inquiry practices such as those of participatory action research.[28] The Just AI approach, discussed in detail in the last chapter, argues that community groups and key stakeholders should be critical collaborators from the earliest phases of project conceptualization. As D'Ignazio and Klein argue, when implemented effectively, just and co-liberatory projects can catalyze significant trust between communities and institutions. Like O'Neal, they argue that community center frameworks offer a better, albeit more challenging, approach to measuring AI fairness. As they write,

> The success of a project designed with co-liberation in mind would also depend on how much trust was built between institutions and communities, how effectively those with power and resources shared their power and resources, how much learning happened in both directions, how much the people and organizations were transformed in the process, and how much inspiration for future work, together, was co-inspired.[29]

These participatory action and co-liberatory frameworks notwithstanding, the general thrust of recommendations for community engagement tend to center on traditional democratic inclusion methods such as public opinion polling[30] and public comment solicitations.[31] At the end of this chapter I will argue that advocates for public inclusion in AI governance would benefit from deeper engagement with the literature on community participation in technical democracy.[32]

Recommendation #3: Regulation/Accountability Earlier in Product Life Cycle

To be blunt, current regulatory structures have been caught flat-footed with respect to AI. Products that cause significant harms to individuals, communities, and the biosphere have proliferated in recent years. Many of these AI systems are released to the market with no significant external scrutiny. Despite the promising tone of the FTC's new guidance, it is clear that this retroactive regulatory approach is expected to continue. Given the long-standing failings of the "do it right or we'll get you later" frameworks, there is a broad consensus among those who advocate for increased regulatory scrutiny of AI that such scrutiny must be deployed earlier in product development. As Data & Society's primer argues, "Much of the processes for obtaining data, aggregating it, making it into digital profiles, and applying it to individuals are corporate trade secrets. This means they are out of the control of citizens and regulators."[33] To intervene effectively and prevent AI from going awry, we need "dynamic (not static) assessment at the start and throughout the AI project lifecycle to account for ongoing decision-making."[34]

The critical importance of early-stage evaluation is central to Tutt's argument for an FDA for AI. He, of course, notes that "Among the most aggressive positions an agency could take would be to require that certain algorithms slated for use in certain applications receive approval from the agency before deployment."[35] While this no doubt seems very aggressive, especially to information/communication technology sector industries that are not used to anything like pre-market approval, it does offer the opportunity to carefully regulate products before broad introduction and subsequent harm. Some of the potential benefits Tutt notes include "conditionally approved subject to usage restrictions—for example, a self-driving car algorithm for cruise control could be approved subject to the condition that it is only approved for highway use. Off-label use of an algorithm, or marketing an unapproved algorithm, could then be subject to legal sanctions."[36]

By and large, Tutt's argument is grounded in a historical understanding of the emergence of the FDA. He makes a compelling argument based on the FDA as a response to so-called snake oil salesmen and champions the FDA in its best incarnation. The way he threads the origins of the FDA with motivating foundations for a new AI regulatory agency is worth looking at in detail. As he argues,

> The arc of the FDA's history shows a relatively stable pattern of public health crises causing the American public to expand the FDA's powers to ensure that drugs are proven safe and effective before they reach the marketplace. Given the close analog between complex pharmaceuticals and sophisticated algorithms, leaving algorithms unregulated could lead to the same pattern of crisis and response. Consequently, we should learn from the FDA's history and decide to act before those crises occur. Some of the world's largest companies are hoping to transform the way people live and work through the power of algorithms. The algorithms of the future may operate in ways that we can neither fully understand nor, without carefully controlled trials, reliably predict. We are poised to enter a world where algorithms can cause similarly outsized risks in similarly difficult-to-know ways as pharmaceutical drugs. Rather than wait for an algorithm to harm many people, we might take the FDA's history as a lesson and instead develop an agency now with the capacity to ensure that algorithms are safe and effective for their intended use before they are released.[37]

As mentioned above, the vision is compelling. But the vision is also anchored in a historic understanding of the FDA that may not effectively capture the current realities of drug and device regulatory practices. Chapter 3's exploration of 510(k) clearance regimes showcases how today's FDA may not serve as an ideal model. Indeed, many argue that the modern incarnation of the FDA is a textbook case of regulatory capture. There is a wealth of scholarship available on how the pharmaceuticals and device industries are regularly able to secure FDA approvals for products of dubious value and significant potential harms.[38] So while an FDA for AI might be a promising solution, it cannot be modeled too closely on today's FDA. Doing so would likely result in Google's ideal vision for a co-governance framework.

RECOMMENDATIONS FOR HEALTH AI GOVERNANCE

The previously discussed recommendations for broad AI govern- ance invoke healthcare and medicine more than they make specific recommendations for health sector policy solutions. That is, health and medicine are broadly recognized as a vibrant area of AI development. And the potential safety concerns of AI-driven medicine are deployed as a key exigency for each vision of AI governance. For example, The European Commission identifies healthcare as a priority sector for AI governance,[39] and the Council of Europe recommendations for reg- ular AI audits indicate the importance of finding sector-specific "ex- pert bodies with responsibilities for overseeing a particular industry (e.g. healthcare) or domain (e.g. autonomous vehicles)."[40] Even Google grudgingly highlights healthcare as one sector where additional regu- lation may be warranted. Of course, they do so in a way they hope will minimize potential regulation for other product lines, recommending "new regulation added only where there is a clear gap and in a way that minimizes overspill," and "sector-specific safe harbor frameworks or li- ability caps."[41]

For the most part, specific attention to the details of health sector reg- ulation focuses on what AI regulation can learn from current or historic drug and device regulatory practices. As mentioned above, Tutt's argu- ment for an FDA for AI is based on the history of FDA drug regulation and enforcement. Similarly, the NSF-funded FEAT Workshop Report argues that non–health sector AI can benefit from an even broader adoption of health governance practices. Specifically, the report authors argue,

> A family who is applying for a home loan does not necessarily need to be taught Machine Learning techniques, but they should be told what the reasons are for the loan being accepted or rejected. This could be patterned after the informed consent process enforced by IRBs; consent forms in the realm of human subjects research must be written at the reading level of the target audience.[42]

Of course, as Chapter 3's discussion of 510(k) clearance outlines, the current FDA model for AI is quite limited and in need of improvement. Cribbing directly from drug and device regulatory agencies without understanding the limits of their current frameworks with respect to AI runs the risk of replicating those limits within a broad AI regulatory framework. Fortunately, researchers in bioethics and health policy are actively working on articulating new foundations for health AI regulation. Scholarship in this area goes a long way toward exposing the limitations of current regulatory frameworks and should be more central to broad AI governance conversations.

Overall, the emerging conversations on health AI governance tend to center on a general commitment to the sense that research ethics are foundational. This is, perhaps, unsurprising given that bioethics, writ large, is primarily grounded in research ethics.[43] The disciplinary origins of bioethics trace back primarily to high-profile cases of research misconduct—the Tuskegee syphilis study, the Stanley Milgram experiments, and the atrocities of Joseph Mengele. As a result, most central bioethical commitments (informed consent, non-maleficence, clinical equipoise) originated in the context of the conduct of ethical recommendations for clinical trials. Additionally, the centrality of ethical clinical research to ethical clinical governance is enshrined in the motivations for the founding of the modern FDA and similar regulatory agencies. In the wake of high-profile events like the thalidomide tragedy, regulatory agencies worldwide adopted new standards for pre-marketing regulation grounded in randomized controlled trials. For example, the 1967 revision to the U.S. Food, Drug, and Cosmetic Act added the requirement for "adequate and well controlled investigations" as part of regulatory scrutiny.[44] Similarly, in 1975, the World Health Organization (WHO) called for all pharmaceutical regulatory agencies to ground marketing approvals in "controlled therapeutic trials."[45] As a result, high-quality clinical research is broadly considered a primary cornerstone for effective and ethical drug and device regulation. This focus on research ethics is echoed in the recent WHO report on ethics and governance for health AI.[46] Similarly, Pascale's *New Laws of Robotics* points to existing professional norms and the oversight capacities of professional medical boards as a primary mechanism for encouraging ethical use of AI.[47] Within this overarching framework, recent work on health AI governance focuses on two primary recommendations for improvement: (1) health AI must demonstrate improvements in health outcomes compared with the current standard of care, and (2) health AI regulation must focus on full product life cycles from preclinical research to post-marketing surveillance.

Recommendation #1: Health AI Must Demonstrate Improvements in Health Outcomes Compared with the Current Standard of Care

In deep medicine, the term "AI chasm" refers to the broad and recurrent gap between high-performing AI systems and real improvements in clinical care. As a recent *Nature Medicine* article puts it, "It is now clear that in silico (computational) validation is not sufficient for successful clinical deployment."[48] A major issue here is overfitting.[49] Overfitting is what happens when an AI's model is so closely tied to the training data that what looks like accurate prediction is almost just memory. When AI models are overfit, they cannot make reliable predictions in new cases. This is why the "platinum standard" mentioned in Chapter 4 requires testing new AI systems on statistically independent data sets. However, researchers are increasingly pointing to the reality that even the platinum standard may not be enough. I'd say we need a "diamond standard" now, but it's all starting to feel too much like airline miles status rankings. As McCradden, Stephenson, and Anderson note, "Accurate predictions within a retrospective, static database do not translate into accurate predictions of health events in a non-stationary clinical context that includes shifting patient trends, operational and/or procedural changes, and practice updates."[50] Similarly, Wu et al. argue that "Evaluating the performance of AI devices in multiple clinical sites is important for ensuring that the algorithms perform well across representative populations. Encouraging prospective studies with comparison to standard of care reduces the risk of harmful overfitting and more accurately captures true clinical outcomes."[51] Clinical outcomes (in addition to model validation) are also central to the FDA's proposed revision to AI regulation.[52] Topol, too, embraces calls for clinical validation of health AI systems, arguing that "the ultimate proof of the clinical utility of AI will come from randomized trials."[53] In a recent interview with *STAT*, he argued that health outcome validation is "the real acid test. You don't want to go forward with something validated [on a computer] and start using it on patients. We know there are all sorts of issues that are different than they are on some pristine, cleaned dataset."[54]

While the AI Chasm is a central motivation of these recommendations, it should not only be understood as a question of innovation adoption. As the next section will describe in more detail, McCradden et al. explicitly center their recommendations in bioethical frameworks that prioritize patient rights, safety, and justice. Additionally, Wu et al.'s article is ultimately aimed at justifying increased regulatory scrutiny. If their recommendations were put into practice, then it would generally take longer to bring devices to market and fewer would qualify. The central concern is assuring that deployed products have been rigorously tested to assure that they are safe and effective. Combining effective tests to assure model validation, clinical effectiveness, and fairness necessarily entails a longer purview of regulatory involvement. Thus, the recommendations to augment AI validation with clinical studies prior to approval invariably lead to recommendations for full–life cycle regulatory scrutiny.

Recommendation #2: Health AI Regulation Must Focus on
Full Product Life Cycles from Preclinical Research to
Post-marketing Surveillance

Regulation of medical devices is generally divided across co-regulatory frameworks. Internal ethics or institutional review boards (ERBs or IRBs) prospectively scrutinize clinical research. In a U.S. context, IRB approval is required to secure FDA approval to use new products in clinical testing. McCradden et al. call for more regular engagement with ERBs as part of preclinical and clinical research. Specifically, they argue that health AI should be rigorously evaluated as part of a three-stage prospective-retrospective clinical trial framework. Their recommended approach begins with exploratory data analysis, subject to ERB/IRB scrutiny with special attention to community engagement, protection of private data, and data governance. At present, Stage 1 is often the entirety of health AI research, and this limitation is largely responsible for the AI chasm. As Topol notes, "There are currently hundreds of published retrospective reports that fall under the rubric of 'clinical trials' of AI, but they are not really trials at all."[55] McCradden et al. also advocate for a silent period where clinical AIs run in the background of hospital data systems and do not report recommendations to clinicians. Stage 2 studies compare the AI's recommendations with provider recommendations in the context of real patient outcomes. Only when the recommendations are found to be effective and fair should an AI device be allowed to proceed to a full clinical trial. Stage 3 recommendations center on superiority trial designs compared with the current standard of care, generalizability, safety, and justice.

Importantly, McCradden et al. recommend that IRBs/ERBs should be involved in pre-study regulation at each stage of the prospective-retrospective trial. The proposed approach also compellingly incorporates ethical and justice reviews, with community approval in Stage 1, fairness in Stage 2, and equity of health outcomes in Stage 3. Ultimately, this may end up being an elegant solution to the challenge of how to include diverse populations in AI research appropriately. If implemented in the right way, Stage 1 could live up to the ideals of Just AI by centering community perspectives in study design. However, Stage 1 must also avoid the harms of using race or racial proxies in algorithmic development. Stages 2 and 3 might then combine to assure that AI recommendations are fair (consistent across demographic categories) and just (do not result in inequitable health outcomes). While I find McCradden et al.'s recommendations very compelling, it is worth noting at this point that IRBs and ERBs are not without their own problems. In a U.S. context, university IRBs sometimes prioritize grant funding over patient health,[56] and there is a disturbing trend of for-profit IRBs, some of which may be little more than pay-for-approval services.[57] For AI-specific improvements to be successfully integrated into ethics reviews, those improvements must be integrated alongside broader system improvements.

When most people think about the proper remit for regulatory agencies like the FDA, the European Medicines Association or the Canadian Therapeutic Products Directorate, they focus on pre-market approval. Pre-market approval processes typically review the results of clinal research in order to determine if products can be brought safely to market and whether they will have the desired effects on patient health. This is an important piece of the overall regulatory puzzle, to be sure, but it is not the end of full–life cycle regulation. In fact, the FDA's proposed Total Product Life Cycle (TPLC) approach for health AI regulation aims to integrate the best practices for machine–learning validation with rigorous safety and efficacy research and post-marketing surveillance; see Figure 7.1. Importantly, the proposed TPLC approach includes not only regulatory review of the research pipeline, but also review of organizational culture for device manufactures. Of course, the devil is always in the details. Reviews of organizational culture have the potential to flag threats to ethics and justice, but the to-be-determined specifics of the regulatory practices will determine if these potential benefits come to pass.

Many agencies also conduct post-marketing surveillance to assure that drugs or devices continue to be safe and effective in broader use cases. At the time of this writing, post-marketing surveillance is gaining increased public attention, as it has caused regulators to pause use of the AstraZeneca

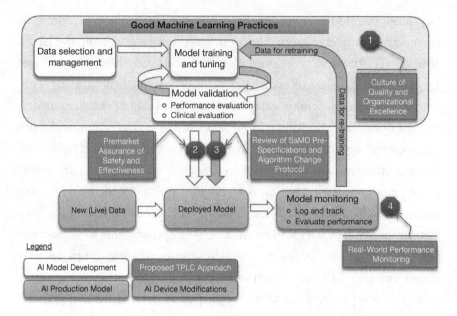

Figure 7.1 The FDA's proposed total product life cycle (TPLC) approach.

and Johnson & Johnson COVID-19 vaccines to evaluate adverse events (blood clots, specifically) in some patients. In their recent proposal for strong regulatory foundations for deep medicine, the FDA has signaled its commitment to maintain a full–life cycle regulatory approach for health AI.[58] See #4 in Figure 7.1. Current FDA regulatory approaches are limited, especially within the context of 510(k) clearances. The FDA does not often become aware of new AI systems until testing is complete, and few 510(k) clearance devices are subject to post-marketing surveillance, an issue that has been recently criticized by Wu et al.[59]

JUST APPROACHES TO REGULATING HEALTH AI

Ultimately, this chapter argues that the parallel conversations on multi-sector and health-specific AI regulation have a lot to say to one another. Establishing a more capacious sense of possible harms is central to both sectors, especially as those in medical contexts work toward more just foundations for bioethics. Robust frameworks for community involvement will be key to these efforts. However, this is one area where health AI scholars offer less detail. On the other hand, since there are already comprehensive regulatory infrastructures for medical devices, researchers in this area have been able to move much more quickly in terms of articulating specific details. McCradden et al.'s three-phase prospective-retrospective trial with its silent phase offers a particularly promising framework for Just and Ethical research in AI more broadly. Imagine if banks had to implement a silent phase for algorithmic credit scoring and report the differences between human and AI recommendations to financial services regulators. This obviously is not going to solve digital redlining overnight, but it would certainly provide a stronger framework for equitable regulation.

Since the broader goal of *The Doctor and the Algorithm* is to focus on deep medicine, most of the rest of this chapter will address how new regulatory proposals might play out in healthcare sectors. In particular, I will discuss two cases where bringing the broad and the narrow regulatory conversations together can potentially improve governance in health AI. In the first case, I will discuss the open question of regulatory Balkanization. Google offers a forceful, if self-serving, argument for dividing regulatory scrutiny into discrete sectors. In what follows, I discuss the limitations of such an approach and one potential U.S.-based model for balancing the needs of domain-specific expertise with coordinated regulatory initiatives. After that, I will close this chapter with some brief remarks about how more effectively to bring community stakeholders into health AI governance.

Regulatory Balkanization

There's an old half-true half-joke about jurisdictional divisions in U.S. regulation. If you're in the freezer aisle of your local grocery store, and you grab a cheese pizza, that pizza's production and marketing will have been regulated by the FDA. Go one freezer case over and grab a pepperoni pizza, and it's a whole different story. Once a pig is involved, so is the U.S. Department of Agriculture (USDA). Now, let's say you like anchovies on your pizza. (Why?!) That pizza is under the jurisdiction of U.S. Fish and Wildlife Service. The U.S. regulatory landscape is largely about fiefdoms. Designated products or sectors are generally under the remit of one specified agency, to the explicit exclusion of other agency concerns. Let's look at a non-joke story about how that plays out.

In 2016, Monsanto sought regulatory approval to introduce a new genetically modified soybean to the market.[60] The new soybean had been engineered specifically to resist a certain pesticide (dicamba). This resistance allows farmers to apply higher quantities of dicamba to their crops with less risk of damage to the soy. Of course, increased pesticide use raises serious concerns about adverse environmental impacts, specifically on local insect populations. Appropriately, Monsanto's new soybean petition went to the USDA, who, as part of their process, solicited public comment. Many individual commenters and environmental organization representatives registered their concern that approval of the new soy variant would lead to deleterious ecosystem impacts. In their response to the public comment, the USDA noted that they were disallowed from considering the pesticide impacts related to approval because that was the purview of the Environmental Protection Agency (EPA). The ironically named Coordinated Framework for Biotechnology Regulation establishes more or less isolated jurisdictional fiefdoms. As a result, the USDA could only consider direct harms brought by the introduction of the plant itself into the environment. Dicamba and dicamba-resistant soy arguably constitute an integrated technology. These seed–pesticide combinations are literally marketed as "crop systems." They are explicitly designed to be used in combination. Yet, here is a case where industry was able to leverage regulatory Balkanization to slice up the pieces of their technological system to secure approval for elements that could be considered "safe" in isolation.

Interestingly, environmental regulation within regulatory agencies may provide a better model for AI regulation. The 1969 National Environmental Policy Act (NEPA) requires federal regulatory agencies to evaluate the environmental impacts of their actions and decisions. Importantly, I am not the first to draw inspiration from NEPA in considering algorithmic governance. Researchers from Data & Society and UCLA Law have drawn inspiration from NEPA's model for impact statements in the development of their approach to "algorithmic impact assessments" or AIAs.[61] My focus here is less on the nature of the assessments themselves than on looking toward NEPA as a model for potential regulatory structures. NEPA requires agencies to conduct environmental impact assessments of regulatory changes not covered by certain limited categorical exclusions. The regulatory framework for these assessments is consistent across agencies. If not covered by a categorical exclusion, then the assessment can either result in a finding of no significant impact (FONSI) or an environmental impact statement (EIS). EISs must be reviewed by final decision-making authorities and included in the record of decision. Importantly, NEPA also established the Council on Environmental Quality, an executive branch office that is responsibility for setting relevant guidelines and maintaining documentation of FONSIs and EISs. In some cases, the Council on Environmental Quality embeds regulators within other agencies to assist with environmental assessments and appropriate reporting. For example, several employees of the Council on Environmental Quality work within different divisions of the FDA to evaluate the potential environmental impacts of new regulations and policies related to food, prescription drugs, and devices. This is not a perfect framework, to be sure. It has been underfunded at times, such that in the FDA, for example, biomedical researchers are sometimes assigned responsibility for evaluating potential environmental impacts. Additionally, the work is largely documentary. The Council on Environmental Quality does not have decision-making authority over individual agencies. Nevertheless, with some sharper teeth, this could be a great model for AI governance. An executive branch Council on Algorithmic Fairness, with embedded agents in sector-specific agencies, could adopt a flexible but coordinated framework for evaluating the potentially adverse impacts of new AI. A strict policy might require a finding of no significant equity impacts (FONSEI, maybe) before a new technology can be approved. A more flexible approach could allow

companies to submit mitigation strategies to be considered alongside equity impact statements.

Community Inclusion

Bringing the people to the table, as it were, is a central thrust of governance proposals in both the broad AI and more narrow health AI purviews.
The European Commission is, perhaps, most forceful in this mandate
where it argues for new regulatory structures that "guarantee maximum
stakeholders participation."[62] While arguments for community inclusion
are a fixture across most AI governance proposals, there is a broad lack of
specificity. Different proposals hint at different potential mechanisms for
community involvement. The WHO points to the potential of citizen science initiatives for supporting early–life cycle community involvement.[63]
The Council of Europe recommends "Member States engage in regular,
inclusive, and transparent consultation with relevant stakeholders—
focusing on the voices of vulnerable groups."[64] While specific details are
not offered in the report, it seems to imply a reliance on fairly standard
governmental mechanisms of stakeholder engagement, e.g., public comment solicitations and advisory panels with community member participation. The FEAT workshop's invocation of participatory action research
suggests a social science orientation to collecting community insights. Jay
Shaw, a scholar of AI health ethics at the University of Toronto, shares this
perspective. During the question-and-answer period at a recent talk, his
advice was, "If you're a ML researcher and you don't know a social science
researcher, go find one!"[65] I'm something of a social scientist myself, and
so I laud this idea, but I'm also mindful that social science research can be
just as extractive as clinical research, prioritizing researcher perspectives
over community values.

When we are talking about either government solicitation of community participation or social science research on community perspectives,
the devil is in the details with respect to the ethics and effectiveness of such
initiatives. In the aforementioned public comment solicitation regarding

Monsanto's new GM soy, it's clear that "public" participation was over-whelmingly dominated by industry groups who were more familiar with the mechanisms of the public comment system.[66] Environmental and anti-GMO advocacy organizations worked to coordinate public comment for its many members and submitted batch comments with short notes with signed letters and short notes from tens of thousands of individuals. However, the USDA evaluation of these comments treated each batch up-load as a single comment, stating that there " '3,716 supported and 941 opposed the use' of dicamba-resistant soybean and cottonseeds (USDA, 2014c, p. 10)."[67] This completely reversed the distribution of community opinions given that there were 32,551 individual Friends of the Earth member commenters and 26,707 individual Center for Food Safety Commenters.[68]

In a similar case of inclusion gone awry, the FDA currently includes consumer and patient representatives on its drug and device advisory committees. These committees help inform regulatory policy and are often called upon to adjudicate complex petitions involving specific drugs or devices. According to the FDA, the role of patient representatives is "to provide direct input to agency staff as they share valuable insight on their experiences with various diseases, conditions, and devices."[69] Unfortunately, designated patient and consumer representatives are also frequently medical experts. My earlier work in this area found that as many as 28% of patient representatives and 78% of consumer repre-sentatives had medical training of some kind.[70] The end result of this is that designated patient and consumer representatives tend to speak on behalf of the clinical experience rather than their patient or consumer experience. In fact, my collaborators found that as the number of pa-tient and consumer representatives at individual meetings increased, the amount of discussion devoted to patient experience or the costs of care actually decreased.[71] Similar research on other FDA patient engagement mechanisms has found those mechanisms to be similarly disappointing in terms of genuine inclusion.[72]

Ultimately, government agencies need serious investments in new approaches that can reliably assure effective public participation in decision-making about technical matters. Fortunately, this work does not need to begin from scratch. There is an entire cottage industry in science and technology studies (STS) and science and technology policy devoted to proposing and assessing robust community inclusion methods. As early as 2005, Gene Rowe and Lynn Frewer identified more than one hundred different proposed mechanisms for public inclusion in science and technology regulation. By analyzing these proposals, they developed a complex typology of public engagement mechanisms and variables. Specifically, they identified the scale of public involvement (communication, consultation, engagement) as well as the primary design variables in public involvement mechanisms (such as participant selection criteria, information dissemination, response modes, medium, etc.). One approach that I keep coming back to is Callon, Lascoume, and Barthe's notion of hybrid forums. The idea of hybrid forums is less about specific policy implications and more about establishing core values for public participation. According to Callon et al., hybrid forums are

> open spaces where groups can come together to discuss technical options involving the collective, hybrid because the groups involved and the spokespersons claiming to represent them are heterogeneous, including experts, politicians, technicians, and laypersons who consider themselves involved. They are also hybrid because the questions and problems taken up are addressed at different levels in a variety of domains, from ethics to economic and including physiology, nuclear physics, and electromagnetism.[73]

Importantly, hybrid forums are hybrid in at least three ways. They are hybrid in the constitution of forum participants (technical experts, community members, regulators). They are hybrid in the purview of discussion (technical matters, economic considerations, equity issues). And they are hybrid in the sense of decision-making authority. Too many regulatory public inclusion mechanisms merely solicit feedback for inclusion in decision-making. The community members do not get a vote on the final decision. As we imagine new and better futures for (health)

AI governance, we need to ensure that proposals center what is known about robust and effective community participation. We need triply hybrid forums.

An important part of Callon et al.'s argument is that community participation is too often delayed to the point of regulatory scrutiny. In fact, they argue that technical democracy becomes more fully hybrid as community members are increasingly involved in problem formation as part of the research collective.[74] Just as there are many proposed mechanisms of communication inclusion in regulatory decision-making, there are many rubrics of community involvement in scientific inquiry. Transdisciplinary research, citizen/community science, and justice-oriented co-labor are three of the most popular. While a full review of these frameworks is beyond the scope of this book, I want to call attention to them as possible resources where we might better flesh out new visions for ethical health AI research. Broadly speaking, clinical research has rigorous standards for conduct and reporting. Multiple governing bodies offer checklists that can be used both as a guide for investigators and as part of review processes. Two popular frameworks are the Consolidated Standards for Reporting of Trials (CONSORT) and Standard Reporting for Interventional Trials (SPIRIT) guidelines. Indeed, McCradden et al. point to the AI extensions of these guidelines (CONSORT-AI and SPIRIT-AI, respectively) as part of their recommendations for prospective-retrospective health AI clinical trials.[75] Unfortunately, the guidelines, as they currently stand, do not offer robust frameworks for community inclusion.[76] The base guidelines each focus considerable attention on appropriate approaches to participation inclusion in trials. The AI extensions add requirements for documenting decisions about data inclusion and exclusion of input data. The SPIRIT base guidelines include requirements regarding describing the "Composition, roles, and responsibilities of the coordinating centre, steering committee, endpoint adjudication committee, data management team, and other individuals or groups overseeing the trial, if applicable." Of course, that "if applicable" suggests that study architects have a great deal of latitude when deciding how or even if they will constitute a community advisory board or include community members on broader trial advisory boards. The CONSORT guidelines have no similar provision. The most robust available framework comes from the lesser-known minimum information about clinical artificial intelligence modeling (MI-CLAIM) guidelines.[77] MI-CLAIM includes a rubric for reproducibility that specifies options for sharing code, third-party fairness audits, and releasing protected versions of the code for public audits. Importantly, MI-CLAIM invites researchers to "choose appropriate tier of transparency" with "tier 4: no sharing" being an acceptable option.[78]

Ultimately, this leads me to a couple of key recommendations for health AI governance with respect to community involvement:

- Clinical trial guidelines like COSORT-AI, SPIRIT-AI, and MI-CLAIM should include clearer language directing health AI researchers to meaningfully engage and account for engagement with community members.
- IRBs and ERBs should formalize their criteria for evaluating community inclusion as part of ethics review. Standards developed should focus on community co-labor and shared decision-making.
- IRBs, ERBs, and regulatory agencies should evaluate and improve their approaches to community representative inclusion to assure that adjudication processes meaningfully engage community member perspectives.

REGULATORY FUTURES

While there is still much work to be done to regulate AI effectively and equitably, I am heartened by the sheer volume of effort in these areas. Scholars, technologists, scientists, policymakers, government boards, and nonprofit organizations the world over are actively working to sketch out new and better regulatory futures. My modest contribution in this area is to argue that, for health, we need to center both the justice commitments of the broad-view and the more fine-grained recommendations of those with sector-specific expertise. In the first case, this means having regulatory frameworks that are oriented toward identifying potential harms in the broadest possible sense. It is no longer acceptable to focus solely on potential harms to target end users. Secondary effects, exploitative uses, and environmental harms must all be part of the puzzle. This work will require sustained engagement with community and stakeholders beyond the limited notion of "stakeholders" so often deployed in industry and regulatory contexts. Prospectively scoping to find communities that may be adversely impacted has to be central to any ethical regulatory regime. And, of course, effectively addressing a more capacious sense of harms across myriad communities will require full–life cycle regulatory involvement. Clearly waiting until products are already out there to intervene is too late, but so, too, is pre-market clearance for mature products. With respect to deep medicine, specifically, bioethicists have already sketched out promising new directions for full–life cycle scrutiny. Through leveraging ERBs/IRBs, enhanced clinical trial guidelines, and new regulatory structures, we have the opportunity to develop an approach to health AI governance that centers patient care and patient outcomes over sales or model performance. As mentioned above, success here will require wedding recommendations for AI governance to broader calls for reform. It's clear that ERBs, IRBs, and agencies like the FDA need to be significantly more independent from the entities they regulate. The details of how to do so are beyond the scope of *The Doctor and the Algorithm*, but they cannot be forgotten as part of recommendations for AI-specific reform.

Finally, to these recommendations, I add my proposals for a NEPA for AI and careful attention to rigorous community engagement through the creation and maintenance of multiple hybrid forums. By combining all of these recommendations, I'm cautiously optimistic that we can achieve a stronger and more ethical second wave of policy implementation. Of course, the second wave cannot be the last wave. Every new refinement will bring new lessons. This is, perhaps, one of the most important reasons why real community engagement must be central to regulatory processes. The people adversely affected by new technologies will be the first to notice when regulatory systems have gone awry. And, so we must create robust systems that allow those most affected to communicate what they know and to be genuinely heard by agencies and regulators.

Conclusion

Just Futures for Deep Medicine

AI is a clear and present danger to health, safety, and equity. AI also has the potential to improve clinical care profoundly. Both of these statements are true, and both are false by dint of their incompleteness. This kind of indeterminacy is a common problem in medicine. Famously, *pharmakon* (the Ancient Greek word at the root of pharmacy) means "drug" but can connote either cure or poison. The Paracelsian maxim that "the dose makes the poison" is likewise a common, albeit misleading, trope of introductory pharmacology. In many ways, AI is a *pharmakon*. It can be both cure and poison. The indeterminacy of a *pharmakon* is inarguably a challenge for medicine, but it does not bring healthcare to a halt. Rather, doctors, researchers, and regulators have slowly built up, over the centuries, systems of checks and balances that ideally lead toward more *pharmakon*-qua-cure than *pharmakon*-qua-poison. Please do not misunderstand me. This has certainly not been some sort of steady progression toward a better world. I am not trying to sell a story about the inevitability of scientific progress. Certainly, there have been plenty of times where medicine went wrong—to borrow a phrase from John Lynch[1]—and continues to go wrong.

Medicine has gone wrong scientifically, ethically, morally, and in terms of justice. The improvements to biomedical research are just as much about hard-fought ethical battles as they are about improvements to scientific

The Doctor and the Algorithm. S. Scott Graham, Oxford University Press. © Oxford University Press 2022.
DOI: 10.1093/oso/9780197644461.003.0009

techniques, per se. Indeed, in the context of clinical trials, it is impossible to separate the ethical from the scientific. Despite all the attention that quality clinical trials get for their scientific rigor, at their core, they respond to moral imperatives. In the U.S. context, clinical research is ostensibly grounded in three moral mandates: respect for persons, beneficence, and justice.[2] These core ethical principles are intended to define and guide human subjects research, including clinical trials. And it is the remit of institutional review boards (IRBs) to assure that researchers stick to these principles. Now, certainly, medicine continues to go wrong in all sorts of ways. It does not unfailingly live up to its ideals. But, of course, we hope that the safeguards of rigorous clinical science, peer review, ethics review, pre-market regulation, post-market surveillance, and even the criminal justice system[3] will stave off the worst of transgressions.

This in mind, it is worth taking stock of exactly where health AI is at this moment. Knowing the strengths and weaknesses of current deep medicine initiatives can help practitioners and advocates alike identify the next best steps toward more just and equitable futures. At the outset of this book, I promised I would address the question of whether or not the AIs of deep medicine qualify as Weapons of Math Destruction (WMDs). According to O'Neil, WMDs are those AI, machine learning, and mathematical systems that lack transparency, rely on surrogate endpoints, and are not updatable.[4] Recidivism prediction is a textbook example of a WMD. These algorithms use survey and court case data on potential parolees to determine their likelihood of reoffending.[5] Parole boards rely on these problematic predictions for release decisions. Recidivism prediction is entirely opaque as proprietary software. It uses surrogate measures, in this case survey results, to make predictions about future behavior. And there is no indication that the algorithm is refined based on follow-up data collection with parolees. In contrast, sabermetrics or moneyball is O'Neil's go-to example for a non-WMD. Home runs, runs, triples, doubles, singles, and walks are the bread and butter of moneyball. A player's ability to round home plate or get on base has a direct and verifiable relationship with winning games. All the data is publicly available, and any predictive algorithms can be easily updated based on the result of new games. As

I mentioned in the Introduction, it is possible that at least some health AI systems are not WMDs. As the preceding chapters have made clear, journal publication and FDA scrutiny are not perfect. However, they may help, in some cases, to provide the kinds of incentives that allow some of these systems to escape the WMD trap. If so, then many of the promises of deep medicine may yet come to pass. With the analyses provided in *The Doctor and the Algorithm*, it is now possible to offer a sort of WMD report card for deep medicine, and that is precisely where I turn next.

WMD REPORT CARD

Identifying WMDs is not a simple exercise in binary classification. There are obvious WMDs (recidivism prediction), and cases that are clearly not WMDs (sabermetrics). However, the WMD-ness of a given health AI can be quite fuzzy. Some of the fully blackboxed and largely unvalidated, untested smartphone apps for e-health are almost assuredly WMDs. Ostensibly custom-tailored, urinalysis-driven in-app vitamin purchases are a huge red flag. However, there are also many examples of well-vetted and published health AI where WMD-ness is a bit harder to pin down. These systems often show some of the features of WMDs (e.g., surrogate endpoint or lack of full code transparency), but those same systems might also embody some of the best recommendations for Ethical or Just AI (e.g., open data or community engaged annotation). Additionally, the details of clinical testing and regulation for deep medicine suggest that identifying WMDs may be somewhat different from those for other consumer technologies. So, before I reflect on the potential WMD status of specific health AI systems, I will first discuss my approach to adapting O'Neil's WMD rubric for the particularities of deep medicine (see Table C.1).

As mentioned above, O'Neil's rubric for WMDs focuses on three primary issues: transparency, surrogacy, and updatability. Much like WMD status itself, none of these are binary categories for health AI. As Table C.1 indicates, transparency can be a function of both commitment to open science principles and of community engagement. Each of these dimensions

Table C.1. O'Neil and Deep Medicine's WMD Rubrics

O'Neil WMDs	Deep Medicine WMDs
Transparency	Openness (Open Science)
	Community Engagement
Surrogacy	Model Validation
	Health Outcomes Assessment
	Trial Design
Updatability	Updatability
—	Hype

comes with its own gradations. Open science can be open data, open code, open access, or all three. Community engagement can be rigorous and full life cycle or all manner of configurations less than that. Community engagement can also be astroturfed. As Benjamin notes, diverse participant recruitment in clinical trials often looks more like user base diversification (i.e., market penetration) than legitimate community engagement.[6] Additionally, model validation can be gold or platinum standard and based on any number of groundtruthing designs. Actual health outcomes assessments are an important part of truly vetting health AI, but the mere presence of health outcomes assessment is not enough to guarantee non-WMD status. Some areas of biomedical research have their own problems with surrogate endpoints.[7] In cancer medicine, you can measure the success of a chemotherapy drug by whether patients live longer or better. Overall survival and quality of life are gold standard measures in oncology. Unfortunately, you can run a faster, cheaper clinical trial by measuring progression-free survival or the amount of time a cancer doesn't appear to get worse.[8] Progression-free survival does not necessarily predict overall survival or quality of life, so it is a dangerous metric to use. Nevertheless, overall survival, quality of life, and similar gold standard metrics are available and broadly used in clinical research. Like home runs, they directly predict the most important results and can be used to create and continuously improve health AI systems. Good metrics must be combined with better trial designs (superiority vs. non-inferiority) in order to decrease the risk of WMD status. Updatability and hype, too, exist on their own continua. Updatability intersects with openness, as fully open systems will be more updatable. Yet, updatability can also be achieved within a blackboxed software system. Finally, promotional language is an ever-present feature of biomedical publication, but at certain thresholds promotion becomes hype. And when hype leads clinicians to put too much faith in expert systems, that surety can bring ruin.

Ultimately, to assure 100% that a given health AI system is not a WMD, one must verify that it (1) is fully open according to open science principles (open data, open code, open access), (2) has rigorous full–life cycle community engagement, (3) uses platinum standard model validation with appropriate and appropriately diverse external data sets, (4) crosses the AI chasm to perform rigorous health outcomes assessments in a well-designed superiority trial that follows from a silent phase, and (5) keeps the hype down to the bare minimums of generic conventions. This is a lot to ask, and many AI developers would balk at these demands. There are probably not more than a handful of systems out there that could possibly meet all these criteria. Still, I would love to see more. Developers in deep medicine absolutely should strive to build systems that meet or exceed each of these guidelines. At the same time, funders, regulators, ERBs/IRBs, and editorial boards should work to incentivize the development of new AI systems that meet these standards. All that said, I am not willing to declare that any system that falls short is surely a WMD. Again, this is not a binary classification problem. In health AI, there is a broad spectrum of system features that combine to determine just how ethical and just a given system is.

To put a little traction on the indeterminacy here, I have prepared a WMD report card for four key systems that were discussed in the preceding chapters. The report card does not so much offer "grades" as describe each system according to its openness, community engagement, model validation, health outcomes assessment, trial design, updatability, and hype risk. The specific systems I have chosen to evaluate were selected to represent the sort of typical range of contemporary deep medicine systems. There are two diagnostic systems: the ProFoundAI™ breast cancer diagnostic system[9] and the onycholysis (toenail fungus) RCNN[10] (each discussed in Chapter 3). There is one digital oracle—the postprandial (post-meal) glycemic responses (PPGR) prediction system—that aims to offer personalized diet advice[11] (addressed in Chapter 2). And I've also evaluated the algorithmic pain prediction (ALG-P), the algorithm pain prediction system designed to offset medical racism[12] (see Chapter 6). Table C.2 provides a snapshot of how each system measures up according to the health AI–specific WMD taxonomy.

Table C.2. WMD Report Card for ProFoundAI™, Onycholysis RCNN, PPGR, and ALG-P

Feature	ProFoundAI™	Onycholysis RCNN	PPGR	ALG-P
Openness	Closed	Open data Open code Open access	Closed	Open data Open code XAI
Community Engagement	Unknown	Unknown	Unknown	Community annotation
Model Validation	Engineered GT Gold standard	Dredged GT Platinum standard (multiple EV sets)	Engineered GT Platinum standard	Forged GT Gold standard
Health Outcomes Assessment	None	None	Surrogate endpoint	None
Trial Design	Non-inferiority	None	Superiority	None
Updatability	Yes (but blackboxed)	Yes, fully open	Unknown	Yes, open data, open code
HypeDx	Promo: 20% Hedge: 10% AUC: 0.852 Risk: low	Promo: 37.5% Hedge: 0% AUC: 0.98 Risk: moderate	Promo: 16.67% Hedge: 0% R: 0.77[a] Risk: low	Promo: 37.5% Hedge 12.5% AUC: 0.861 Risk: high

NOTE: EV = external validation.
[a]The PPGR is a predictive (rather than classification system), thus performance is measured not with AUC but based on the correlation between predicted and measured glycemic response.

Ultimately, each of these systems has elements that would prevent it from being immediately classified as a WMD. ProFoundAI™ is tested in a real clinical context. It is updatable, and it has a relatively low hype risk score. Onycholysis RCNN is an exemplar of open science with accessible data and code. It is also published in an open access journal and uses platinum standard validation with multiple external validation sets. PPGR is the only system in the table with a health outcomes assessment and a superiority trial, and it is at very low risk of hype. Finally, ALG-P uses community ground truth annotation and has both open data and open code.

At the same time, all four systems have issues that might raise some concern. ProFoundAI™ is a fully closed system and was tested using the minimal non-inferiority threshold for 510(k) clearance. Despite being open access, the Onycholysis RCNN data set is not particularly diverse, and the study offers no health outcomes assessment. What's more, it is pushing the threshold for high-risk of hype with an abstract that is 37.5% promotional. PPGR does not participate in any dimension of open science, it has no known community engagement protocols, and the health outcomes assessment focuses on a surrogate endpoint (glycemic response) that has a complex relationship to target health outcomes. Finally, ALG-P has no external validation set, offers a problematic construct for patient trust in the context of inequity, and uses eXplainable AI (XAI) frameworks that may be less accurate or induce more clinician trust than unexplainable systems. ALG-P is also in the highest risk zone for hype with nearly 40% promotional language, credibility-bolstering hedges, and a less-than-outstanding area under the curve (AUC) score.

Reviewing Table C.2, two areas stick out as being in the greatest need of improvement: (1) there is an unfortunate lack of health outcomes assessments and quality clinical trials, and (2) community engagement is one of the most poorly represented categories. As discussed in the previous chapter, the former is well recognized as an immediate cause for concern in deep medicine and bioethics alike. Proposals for three-stage clinical trials[13] and newly promulgated reporting standards[14] all point toward a new era of health AI that moves away from an overreliance on in silico validation alone. Importantly, even the most enthusiastic advocates for health AI are on board with this transition. Recent collaborative publications featuring Eric Topol have argued for rigorous health outcomes assessments in deep medicine broadly[15] and dietary AI specifically,[16] and he is a core member of the minimum information about clinical artificial intelligence modeling (MI-CLAIM) standards development team.[17] While those in critical algorithm studies, broadly conceived, certainly recognize the need for deeper community engagement in AI, demands for community-centered research are also central to conversations about just and ethical futures in health research beyond AI. This suggests to me that we need more efforts to incentivize thorough community involvement. IRBs, ERBs, and government regulators can help here, but that is all stick. Some additional carrot is probably in order. Fortunately, there are a few emerging developments in this area that might pave the way for better futures in deep medicine. Since improvements for research frameworks in deep medicine are already well in hand and being spearheaded by more appropriate experts, I will focus more of *The Doctor and the Algorithm* on emerging incentives for community-led development.

Before I do, however, it is worth noting the limitations of this analysis. Here I have attended to whether or not a few specific well-researched and published health AI technologies might be at risk of being WMDs. As discussed in Chapter 5, accounts of specific systems are generally at only a moderate risk for hype. The biggest dangers for the future of health AI come from problematic meta-discourse, including both (1) systematic reviews that are built on overly optimistic or unrepresentative collections of studies and (2) the techno-evangelism that fuels venture capitalism. When discussions about AI are taken away from the specific contexts of vetting a given system, they tend to transition quickly into the realm of technochauvinism as exhibited in Chapter 2. Unbridled enthusiasm for oracular AI frequently gives way to a misplaced surety and an unfortunate willingness to embrace less ethical technological configurations. The best hope for the future of deep medicine is to keep it grounded in steady research on individual systems, to keep it anchored in rigorous research practices guided by effective ethical oversight, and to keep it led by the communities most likely to be adversely affected by new technologies.

COMMUNITY-LED DEVELOPMENT

As mentioned previously, researchers in medicine and public health are increasingly recognizing the importance of (social determinants of health) SDoH.[18] The long-standing biomedical model tends to focus clinical attention on biological phenomena (genetics, medical history) and individual behavior (choices about diet, exercise, and work–life balance). A SDoH framework recognizes that social configurations including systemic inequities have huge impacts on overall health, both directly and indirectly by circumscribing an individual's available choices. Environmental and economic injustices often combine to produce severe health inequities. On an environmental injustice front, poor and minoritized communities are more likely to be the victim of industrial waste dumps and less likely to be prioritized for lead pipe and paint remediation. Economic injustice often leads to intractable food deserts where access to healthy food is greatly curtailed. For someone working 60 hours a week at two part-time jobs, an hour-long bus ride to a full-scale supermarket is often just not in the cards. Factor in the relatively high costs of fresh fruits and vegetables, and it starts to become patently dishonest to describe this individual's foodways as "choice." One poignant example where environmental, economic, and health injustice all come together is the "obesocarcinogenic environment."[19] Emerging evidence indicates that there are significant and underdiscussed relationships between cancer and obesity-related illness. The latest findings point toward physiological mechanisms that can result in a situation where obesity encourages cancer growth and development.[20] Importantly, these are complex mechanisms intimately tied up in socioeconomic disparities and SDoH. Environmental and economic injustices combine to produce situations that fuel obesity and cancer rates in impoverished communities. Obesity and cancer comorbidity and risk coincidence are further exacerbated by health injustices that limit screening and treatment options for members of poor and minoritized communities.[21]

In these kinds of complex, multicausal situations, justice-oriented interventions require transdisciplinary research that effectively coordinates the efforts and expertises of biomedical researchers, social scientists, and community leaders.[22] Unfortunately, even in research that centers on SDoH, this not a common model. Take, for example, a new SDoH-focused AI system developed by the University of Virginia (UVA) Health System. This project begins in a good place, centered on SDoH. As Amy Salerno, one of the UVA project leaders, notes, "Industry-wide and society-wide, there's a lot more recognition of the social determinants of health. In Charlottesville specifically, we've been looking at inequities and disparities in our local community and among our patients, and noting the tie to health outcomes."[23] An increasing focus on SDoH, combined with a recognition that current healthcare and healthcare IT infrastructures do not effectively support data collection related to SDoH, led UVA to a great idea—collecting SDoH information directly from unstructured clinician notes in electronic health records (EHRs). The resulting natural language processing system mines the free text entry part of UVA's electronic health records and looks for information related to SDoH that might inform clinical decision-making. As far as I can tell, this is a good project, and I am glad it exists. However, it is not community led in an ideal transdisciplinary way. SDoH information is invariably filtered through clinical judgment. Only when clinicians choose to capture this information as a part of their notes will the AI system have a chance at processing it and using it to inform clinical decision-making or public health effectively. Unfortunately, this is another stopgap system like ALG-P. It folds community-centered information into the dominant logics of clinical medicine to be mined, datafied, and re-presented according to clinical sensibilities about information utility.

Broadly speaking, there are two serious limitations to this kind of intervention from a transdisciplinary/Just AI perspective: (1) As mentioned above, it reduces SDoH data to the perspectives of clinicians/researchers, and (2) it assumes that the best solutions will come from outside affected communities. Too much of SDoH research is built on an extractive research paradigm. It assumes that when outsider-experts can effectively capture SDoH information, those outsider-experts will be able to effectively intervene. Simply put, there is no substitute for the lived reality of

SDoH when it comes to identifying possible solutions. Indeed, members of socioeconomic-disparities communities have been navigating and developing mitigation strategies for those SDoH their entire lives. More importantly, most communities have embedded community organizations replete with community experts who are likely to have the best insights into both the complexities of a target problem and possible solutions. Outside perspectives can be helpful, but they cannot be offered acontextually. This is why community-led transdisciplinary methodologies are routinely offered as the most just approach.

While this is not the dominant paradigm for SDoH research, there is some good news, in terms of new incentives from the NIH. Recently, the NIH Common Fund (the coordinating center for capacious cross-institute research) has launched the Bridge2AI program. A central initiative of Bridge2AI is to fund the creation of community-centered data sets built according to the best practices of Ethical AI. Diverse team building is a central commitment of the program. Often, in biomedical research contexts, diversity is reduced to either participant recruitment or workforce development. These are both important initiatives, but obviously not the sum total of ways to define diversity. The Bridge2AI program description has a remarkably expansive and heartening list of configurations that qualify as diverse team building. They include the typical foci on diversifying the biomedical workforce, but also:

- Transdisciplinary collaborations that require unique expertise and/or solicit diverse perspectives to address research questions.
- Inclusion of community-based partners to ensure alignment of research goals and activities with community values.[24]

At the time of this writing, the Bridge2AI program is newly announced, so it remains to be seen how many of the funded projects will operationalize diversity according to transdisciplinary or Just AI principles. Regardless, I expect that programs like Bridge2AI will proliferate in the next few years, and this is a cause for genuine, if cautious, optimism.

JUST AND ETHICAL FUTURES

Ultimately, cautious optimism is where I hope to end *The Doctor and the Algorithm*. Certainly, this book and the collected work of critical algorithm studies and justice-oriented bioethics have shown that deep medicine warrants careful skepticism. Yet the coordinated efforts of Ethical AI, Just AI, and AI-focused bioethics are having a real and observable impact on the practice and regulation of deep medicine. As mentioned in Chapter 7, core recommendations for a more ethical deep medicine argue that (1) health AI must demonstrate improvements in health outcomes compared with the current standard of care, and (2) health AI regulation must focus on full product life cycles, from preclinical research to post-marketing surveillance. Proposals for the three-phase clinical trial and related reporting standards are promising developments in this area. Additionally, as I have argued in this book, these efforts can be meaningfully and substantively improved through more coordination between advocates of Ethical AI and bioethicists who attend to deep medicine. Health AI will always occupy a medial position between computer science and medicine. Thus, the best foundation for ethical medicine will require carefully calibrating the insights of ethics experts in each area. To that end, bioethics recommendations for health AI improvements must be combined with Ethical AI's commitments to transparency and auditability. Open science principles can help here, as I argued in Chapter 3. But, of course, the work must be done carefully. Not all insights of Ethical AI writ large are perfectly attenuated to the demands of deep medicine. For example, Ethical AI's commitment to transparency often focuses on XAI, which can lead to underperforming systems and misplaced trust.[25] Nevertheless, I am optimistic that these two areas can be brought more fully into conversation with one another. Indeed, that has been a major aim of *The Doctor and the Algorithm*. If the combined recommendations of ethical experts in both areas take hold in health AI, then we have a real shot at a more ethical foundation for deep medicine.

Unfortunately, the recent history of self- and co-regulatory governance models has clearly shown that the tech industry simply will not voluntarily commit to ethical AI. Industry investments in ethical development will have to be guaranteed by effective regulatory structures. Fortunately, governments and regulatory agencies in both EU and U.S. contexts are actively working on new governance frameworks for AI. In the best cases, new regulatory initiatives will respond to the core recommendations of AI governance advocates. Specifically, new frameworks must (1) be attuned to a more expansive sense of possible harms, (2) center community and stakeholder groups in governance and regulatory decision-making, and (3) increase regulatory scrutiny throughout full product life cycles. For the most potentially dangerous sectors, this will likely require rigorous pre-market approval of new AI technologies. A so-called FDA for AI is a common proposal here, and certainly I agree that effective AI regulation will require the coordinated efforts of relevant technical and ethical experts. In the last chapter, I proposed a more diffuse approach modeled on the National Environmental Policy Act (NEPA). Specifically, I think the best regulatory model may involve a central executive branch Council on Algorithmic Fairness, with embedded agents in sector-specific agencies. Regulatory decisions should be preceded by careful study of the potential equity impacts, and at the very least mitigation measures must be required.

One of the biggest criticisms of the FDA is that it does not do its own research. That is, pharmaceutical companies conduct their own clinical trials and submit the results to the FDA for approval. Currently, the same thing happens with respect to NEPA scrutiny of new drug approvals. Unfortunately, this can lead to poorly designed ecotoxicology studies where drug companies test the ecosystem impacts of their products at concentrations that are much lower than those observed in the environment. This simply cannot be allowed to happen with health AI. Fortunately, even well-conducted AI audits are much cheaper and less time consuming than drug trials or even laboratory ecotoxicology. A NEPA for AI could maintain its own closed repositories of clinical data and use that data to test the differential equity impacts of newly proposed AI systems. By keeping the data and the testing closed off from industry, companies would find it harder to put their thumb on the scales, as it were.

Importantly, an ethical future for deep medicine is not necessarily the same thing as a just future. Racism, ableism, sexism, and other structural inequities continue to be a significant part of Western medicine, bio-medical research, and clinical care. A just future for AI, a just future for medicine, and a just future for health AI will require more substantive changes. Ethical recommendations tend to lean into clinical science. They rightly argue that new clinical interventions must be rigorously tested so that providers can be sure that care is best suited to the medical needs of patients. Clinical research can do amazing things, but it absolutely cannot do everything. The best methods of randomized controlled trials are simply not well suited to understanding structural inequities. Insights from sociology, anthropology, political science, economics, communica-tion, rhetoric, critical race theory, and the humanities broadly must all be brought meaningfully into the conversation. I would echo again Jay Shaw's exhortation to health AI researchers: "If you're a ML researcher and you don't know a social science researcher, go find one!"[26] Of course, as I mentioned in the last chapter, these conversations cannot be exclu-sively led by academic frameworks and perspectives. A just approach to dismantling health injustice will require following the lead of those most impacted by systemic inequities. In health AI, community-guided and community-led research will be a critical part of problematic academic saviorism. Consider the ethical challenges presented by ALG-P, the os-tensible racism mitigation AI algometer described in Chapter 6. The most affected community members were involved in the study in an impor-tant way. They provided critically important annotations for the training data. That said, I am not sure how broadly Black patients would support a system that technologically "verifies" pain reports, as such a system seems to replicate long-standing patterns of clinical distrust of Black pain.

It is with this context in mind that I recommended a more precau-tionary approach to AI development, one that centers on community perspectives at the outset. Specifically, in Chapter 6, I recommended that those who wish to offer technological solutions to health inequity should, at the very least, address these questions: (1) Is the proposed intervention likely to address an unmet or under-met community need substantially?

(2) Have members of the communities most likely to be affected by the intervention been substantively involved in project conceptualization, putative benefits, risk assessment, data curation, and training set labeling? (3) Does the project team have a robust plan for evaluating unintended consequences during design, development, testing, and distribution? (4) Does the project team have a robust plan for supporting long-term community-centered justice-oriented initiatives in this area? Without a clear yes to each of these questions, researchers are in dodgy ethical territory if they proceed with research and development. Fortunately, programs like the NIH's Brigde2AI provide one possible model for encouraging research that can answer affirmatively to these questions.

Unfortunately, many will proceed anyway. Technochauvinism is generally a death blow to precaution. As Broussard has compellingly argued, the cultures of academic computer science and Silicon Valley do much to encourage privileged "experts" to forge headlong into misguided and ethically dubious initiatives.[27] Medicine, of course, often finds itself caught up in a similar kind of biomedical chauvinism. Unethical clinical research is frequently well rewarded. Saul Krugman received a number of prestigious awards for his research intentionally infecting disabled children with hepatitis at the Willowbrook School.[28] Biomedical researchers and their sponsoring institutions can also be highly recalcitrant in the face of ethical oversight. Eugene Senger and the University of Cincinnati were quick to decry congressional scrutiny of their DOD-sponsored whole body radiation experiments as "political" interference into objective scientific decision-making.[29] Largely, this recalcitrance was successful at keeping ethical scrutiny behind closed doors. This is a prima facie example of why community groups need to be more fully involved in both internal governance and external regulatory processes. Just and Ethical oversight needs to be guided by forums that are fully hybrid in terms of expertise, remit, and decision-making authority. As I mentioned in the previous chapter, researchers in science and technology policy can be a guide here (e.g., Callon, Barthe, and Lascoumes).[30] Of course, sector-specific expertise will remain essential to these efforts. It would be unhelpful to simply drop a community governance model developed for climate change into a health AI context. In much the same way that Ethical AI and clinical bioethics need careful coordination, science and technology policy recommendations will have to be carefully attenuated to the sector-specific needs of health justice.

There is much promise in deep medicine, and that promise is usually articulated in terms of system performance or potential improvements to health outcomes. However, for me, the greatest promise for health AI comes from the enthusiastic and engaged work of its careful critics. I am not really sure it's fair to describe AI as "delayed" in medicine, but to the extent that it is, that delay has done the world a favor. The dangerous AIs of social media, consumer finance, and predictive policing were ushered in on a wave of techno-utopian rhetoric. In the early days of Web 2.0, it still seemed vaguely plausible that the Internet might live up to some of its utopian hype. That misguided optimism has been appropriately left aside, and technologists, bioethicists, social scientists, and humanists are embracing deep medicine with an intentional critical posture. And it is making a difference. The work of leading-edge scholars like Ruha Benjamin, Cathy O'Neil, Safyia Noble, Meredith Broussard, Timnit Gebru, and many others has encouraged a broadly critical approach to AI. Society is paying attention. Governments are paying attention. Even though this work was not focused particularly on the clinical contexts of AI, it has created a situation where the embrace of AI in medicine can be met with more mature critical tools. Accordingly, scholars like Melissa McCradden, Jay Shaw, and Alex John London are working to help ensure that AI's progress in medicine is carefully shaped by the best insights of Ethical and Just AI. As a result, calls for better research methods abound. Proposals for more rigorous AI regulation are proliferating across jurisdictions and national contexts. None of this means it is time to be complacent. There is still much work to done. But if we can capitalize on this momentum to help assure that we really are at the outset of a new, well-regulated, rigorously validated, and community-led era for deep medicine, then I, for one, am looking forward to the next phase of health AI.

A.1. BEARING CAPACITY SIMULATION

This portion of the appendix describes the technical details behind the bearing capacity simulations presented in Chapter 4. In what follows, I detail my approach to data and feature selection, modeling, simulating engineered ground truth, and simulating forged ground truth simulation.

A.1.2. Data Set and Feature Selection

For all ground truth simulations, I used the canonical Wisconsin Breast Cancer Dataset (WBCD). The WBCD provides diagnostic information on fine-needle aspirant slides of possible breast cancer cells. A pathologist visually evaluated each slide and graded the cells according to several categories, including bare nuclei, cell shape, marginal adhesion, and so forth. Each slide was rated on a scale of 1 to 10 for each category, with 1 being normal and 10 being highly abnormal. The cells on each slide are also classified as either benign or malignant. The complete WBCD includes data on 569 slides. In order to prepare these data for training and testing in the simulations, I first set aside 100 cases for use in subsequent validation and secondary modeling. I also rebalanced the remaining data set to ensure that there was an equal number of benign and malignant cases. This left 478 cases for initial AI training. Since the goal of the bearing capacity simulation was to develop 500 classifiers with different levels of performance, I used both a very small number of variables and a small sample size for training. Each classifier was trained on a random sample of 10 cases, using only the values for cell shape and marginal adhesion. Each of the individual grading categories in the WBCD is highly predictive of malignancy, so it is possible to train a reasonably performant classifier on a small subset of features. This was the primary aim of the article discussed in Chapter 1.[1] The article used rough set theory to identify the smallest number of features that would produce the most effective model performance.

A.1.2. Model Architectures

All models used in the bearing capacity simulations were trained using R's caret[2] library deployed on a desktop workstation (Dell G5, core i3-9300, 16 GB RAM). All models were neural networks. In order to induce more variability in classifier performance, I set the code to generate values randomly for the number of hidden layers and the weight decay as part of fitting each model. In many cases AIs are trained using random number seeding and pre-specified sampling protocols (e.g., bootstrapping or k-fold cross validation). I did not set any of these parameters in the bearing capacity simulation. The intent and result of this were to foster additional variability in baseline model performance. With carefully controlled sampling protocols and hyperparameters, each replication of the simulation would produce identical pairs of models. This would eliminate the possibility of meaningful performance comparisons across model pairings. With this variability and lack of tuning, only 499 of the attempted 500 models fit and were able to make predictions about potential malignancy.

A.1.3. Engineered Ground Truth Simulation

To simulate engineered ground truth, I used the 499 trained models to predict the classification (malignant or benign) of the reserved 100 cases. I used an identical modeling approach to train 499 new classifiers on a training set composed of the first 50 of the 100 reserved cases. The second set of classifiers were trained using the first set's predictions as the training labels. I then used the second set of models to predict classifications for the remaining 50 cases in the test set. This method provided 499 pairings of classifiers, each with a known accuracy value for the original model (proxy for a lab test with a known accuracy), a reportable accuracy for the second model (relative to first model predictions), and a true accuracy (relative to known ground truth from the original WBCD).

A.1.4. Forged Ground Truth–Bearing Capacity Simulation

To conduct the forged ground truth–bearing capacity simulation, I selected 200 random pairings of the initial 499 classifiers. Predictions on the reserved 100 sample were reconciled based on consensus for malignancy. That is, if both classifiers agreed that the case was malignant, then it was classified as malignant. In the case of either disagreement or both agreeing that the case was benign, it was classified as benign. The forged ground truth simulation compares the inter-rater reliability of the two systems to the accuracy of the consensus predictions (measured against actual ground truth per the WBCD).

A.2. HYPEDX AND HEDGEDX

This section of the Appendix describes the development of the HypeDx and HedgeDx parsers. In what follows, I detail the approach to groundtruthing,

feature engineering, model development, and benchmarking. I also provide some additional details on the statistical analyses presented in
Chapter 5.

A.2.1. Groundtruthing

The HypeDx and HedgeDx systems were designed to identify promotional and hedged claims about AI systems in biomedical discourse. To
prepare a training set for HypeDx, abstracts were collected for each of
the 82 studies explored in Liu et al.'s meta-analysis.[3] These abstracts were
tokenized by sentence, creating a complete data set of 938 sentences that
would be used for training and validation. For groundtruthing, each of
these sentences was coded by two human raters according to three coding
categories: (1) neutral claim, (2) promotional claim, and (3) hedged claim.
A description of each of these codes and the criteria for non-claim are
available in Table A.1. All categories are binary, and each sentence was
coded for presence or absence of markers related to the claim type. Given
this approach, it is possible for claims to have both promotional and
hedged elements, but it is not possible for claims to be neutral and have
more than one category.

Initial annotation was completed on a subsample of 288 abstract
sentences. Annotations were applied independently by each rater, and
interrater reliability was assessed using Cohen's kappa. Initial κ values
were fair to good, with accuracy scores of 92%–95.1%. The two raters used
these results to conduct a norming exercise where they discussed points of
disagreement. They then re-coded the 288 sentences independently, along
with an additional 650 sentences to create the final n = 938 sentences
training and validation data set. Final interrater reliability by coding category is as follows:

- Neutral claim: κ = .705, accuracy 93%, substantial agreement[4]
- Hedged claim: κ = .673, accuracy 93.9%, substantial agreement
- Promotional claim: κ = .811, 94%, almost perfect agreement

Table A.1. CODING CATEGORIES FOR GROUNDTRUTHING HYPEDX AND HEDGEDX.

Code	Description
Neutral Claim	Claim about AI working or not working. Simple declarative statements. *Example:* The AI (ensemble model; ResNet-152 + VGG-19 + feedforward neural networks) results showed test sensitivity / specificity / AUC values of (96.0 / 94.7 / 0.98), (82.7 / 96.7 / 0.95), (92.3 / 79.3 / 0.93), (87.7 / 69.3 / 0.82) for the B1, B2, C, and D data sets.
Promotional Claim	Claim about AI that includes promotional language (significantly, better, impressive, favorable comparison to humans) *Example:* By training with a data set comprising 49,567 images, we achieved a diagnostic accuracy for onychomycosis using deep learning that was superior to that of most of the dermatologists who participated in this study.
Hedged Claim	Claim about AI that includes hedges (moderately, suggests, might indicate, non-significant, approaching significant). *Example:* Receiver operating characteristic analysis revealed non-significant differences (p-values 0.45–0.47) in the AUC of 0.84 (DLS), 0.88 (experienced and intermediate readers) and 0.79 (inexperienced reader).
Non-Claim	Not a claim or not about evaluated AI. *Example:* The validation data sets comprised 100 and 194 images from Inje University (B1 and B2 data sets, respectively), 125 images from Hallym University (C data set), and 939 images from Seoul National University (D data set).

Ultimately, these results were reliable enough to form a training set for the HypeDx and HedgeDx parsers. Annotation disagreements were adjudicated by a third rater (me), and then processed for feature engineering.

A.2.2. Feature Engineering

For both the HypeDx and the HedgeDx systems, parts-of-speech (POS) average (aveloc) proved to be the most reliable and performant approach to feature engineering. I developed the POS aveloc method to provide a syntactically focused feature engineering option.[5] To implement this approach, I used the popular spaCy natural language processing toolkit. spaCy, itself, is an example of machine learning and text classification. It applies "learned" insights from large textual corpora to identify POS or named entities. POS aveloc feature engineering occurs in two steps: (1) the text of interest is parsed to identify parts-of-speech, and (2) the average location (within each sentence) of each part of speech is identified. For this project, I used spaCyr,[6] a library that provides an interface between a python implementation of spaCy language models and an R development environment. Tables A.2 and A.3 detail the two steps of POS aveloc feature engineering on a sample sentence from the data set.

A.2.3. Model Architectures

Both HypeDx and HedgeDx were trained with the R caret package[7] using a random 80/20 train/test split and 10-fold cross-validation with 5 repeats. I tested Neural Network, Naive Bayes, K-Nearest Neighbor, and bagged Classification and Regression Trees (CART). The bagged CART models had the highest accuracy for both the HypeDx and HedgeDx models at AUC = 0.8947 and AUC = 0.8012, respectively. The ROC curves for the final models are available in Figure A.1. All feature extraction and modeling were performed on a desktop workstation (Dell G5, core i3-9300, 16 GB RAM).

A.2.4. Statistical Analyses

Correlation tests were performed with Spearman's rank correlation coefficient due to the non-normality of the data. Categorical comparisons

Table A.2. POS AVELOC STEP 1 spaCY PART-OF-SPEECH TAGGING WITH ADJECTIVES (ADJ) HIGHLIGHTED.

ID	Token	POS
1	To	PART
2	develop	VERB
3	a	DET
4	deep	ADJ
5	convolutional	ADJ
6	neural	ADJ
7	network	NOUN
8	(	PUNCT
9	DCNN	PROPN
10	)	PUNCT
11	that	DET
12	can	VERB
13	automatically	ADV
14	detect	VERB
—	—	—

NOTE: Input text: To develop a deep convolutional neural network (DCNN) that can automatically detect laryngeal cancer (LCA) in laryngoscopic images.

Table A.3. POS AVELOC STEP 2 AVERAGE LOCATION PER SENTENCE IDENTIFICATION WITH (ADJ) HIGHLIGHTED.

ADJ_ave_loc	ADP_ave_loc	ADV_ave_loc	DET_ave_loc	NOUN_ave_loc
7.5	20	13	7	16.5

were evaluated using the estimation statistics framework. Two-group and shared-control estimation plots were used to compare promotional proportions and maximum AUC scores by category. Shared-control estimation plots are part of the estimation statistics framework recently promulgated as a robust alternative to null-hypothesis significance testing.[8] Estimation plots focus analytic attention on population parameters, mean differences, and effect sizes over p-values. The approach here uses Efron's technique for bias-corrected accelerated bootstrap (BCa) estimation to

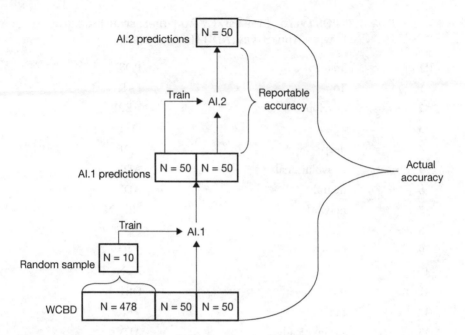

Figure A.1. Representative POS aveloc feature engineering highlighting average adjective location.

account for skewed populations.[9] Each analysis ran 5,000 BCa iterations to derive mean difference estimates within 95% confidence intervals.

INTRODUCTION

1. Eric Topol, Deep Medicine: How Artificial Intelligence Can Make Healthcare Human Again (New York: Basic Books, 2019).
2. Topol, *Deep Medicine*, 5.
3. I'm certainly painting with an overly broad brush here, and it's worth noting that no single book fits purely into one of these three categories. Topol has an obligatory chapter on the dangers of deep medicine. Most contributions to critical algorithm studies have a section on how future work in AI might be channeled for good (or at least not bad).
4. Thomas Mullaney, "Your Computer Is on Fire," in Your Computer Is on Fire, ed. Thomas Mullaney et al. (Cambridge, MA: The MIT Press, 2021), 3.
5. Ibid., 6.
6. Topol, *Deep Medicine*, 4.
7. Lei Xing, Maryellen L. Giger, and James K. Min, eds., Artificial Intelligence in Medicine: Technical Basis and Clinical Applications (London: Academic Press, 2021).
8. Efstahios D. Gennatas and Jonathan H. Chen, "Artificial Intelligence in Medicine: Past, Present, and Future," in *Artificial Intelligence in Medicine*, 9.
9. Daniel Zeng, Zhidong Cao, and Daniel B. Neill, in *Artificial Intelligence in Medicine*, 438.
10. Nic Fleming, "How Artificial Intelligence Is Changing Drug Discovery," *Nature 557* (2018): s55–s57.
11. David H. Freedman, "Hunting for New Drugs with AI," *Nature 576* (2019): s50–s53.
12. "BPM31510," Berg Health, n.d., https://www.berghealth.com/research/healthcare-professionals/pipeline/bpm31510/.
13. Topol, *Deep Medicine*, 12.
14. Ibid., 80.
15. Ibid., 164.
16. Mullaney, "Your Computer," 3.
17. Ruha Benjamin, Race after Technology: Abolitionist Tools for the New Jim Code (Cambridge: Polity Press, 2019).

18. Safiya Umoja Noble, Algorithms of Oppression: How Search Engines Reinforce Racism (New York: New York University Press, 2018).

19. Ibid., 3.

20. Benjamin, *Race after*, 5–6.

21. Ibid., 143.

22. Ibid., 88.

23. Cathy O'Neil, Weapons of Math Destruction: How Big Data Increases Inequality and Threatens Democracy (New York: Crown, 2016).

24. Ibid., 3.

25. Topol, *Deep Medicine*, 158.

26. Ibid., 177–178,

27. Kelly M. Hoffman et al., "Racial Bias in Pain Assessment and Treatment Recommendations, and False Beliefs about Biological Differences between Blacks and Whites," *PNAS 113*, no. 16 (2016): 4296–4301.

28. Benjamin, *Race after*, 154.

29. Ibid., 154–155.

30. O'Neil, *Weapons*, 17–19.

31. Food and Drug Administration, Guidance for Industry and FDA Staff: Statistical Guidance on Reporting Results from Studies Evaluating Diagnostic Tests, March 13, 2007, https://www.fda.gov/media/71147/download.

32. John Lynch et al., "Bridging Science and Journalism: Identifying the Role of Public Relations in the Construction and Circulation of Stem Cell Research among Laypeople," *Science Communication 36*, no. 4 (2014): 479–501; 482.

33. "Technochauvinism" is the overly enthusiastic embrace of technological innovation as the cure for all of society's ills. Technochauvinists hope the tech fix will offer a panacea that avoids the hard work of pursuing social justice. See Meredith Broussard, Artificial Unintelligence: How Computers Misunderstand the World (Cambridge, MA: The MIT Press, 2019).

34. Catherine D'Ignazio and Lauren F. Klein, Data Feminism (Cambridge, MA: MIT Press, 2020).

CHAPTER 1

1. In the episode "The Naked Now," audiences are told that Data has a fully functional sexual anatomy and that he's even "programmed in multiple techniques, a broad variety of pleasuring"; *Star Trek: The Next Generation*, "The Naked Now," #40271-103, episode 3, written by D.C. Fontana and Gene Roddenberry, June 1987.

2. Efstahios D. Gennatas and Jonathan H. Chen, "Artificial Intelligence in Medicine: Past, Present, and Future," in *Artificial Intelligence in Medicine: Technical Basis and Clinical Applications*, ed. Lei Xing, Maryellen L. Giger, and James K. Min (London: Academic Press, 2021), 5.

3. Benjamin, *Race after*, 41.

4. Bruno Latour, Science in Action: How to Follow Scientists and Engineers through Society (Cambridge, MA: Harvard University Press, 1987), 2–3.

5. Latour, *Science*, 131.

6. Halcyon Lawrence, "Siri Disciplines," in Your Computer Is on Fire, ed. Thomas Mullaney et al. (Cambridge, MA: The MIT Press, 2021), 179.

7. Bruno Latour, Pandora's Hope: Essays on the Reality of Science Studies (Cambridge, MA: Harvard University Press), 183.

8. S. Scott Graham, The Politics of Pain Medicine: A Rhetorical-Ontological Inquiry (Chicago: University of Chicago Press), 123.

9. Latour, Science, 137.

10. Catherine D'Ignazio and Lauren F. Klein, Data Feminism (Cambridge, MA: MIT Press), 8.

11. D'Ignazio and Klein, Data, 53.

12. Benjamin, Race after, 78.

13. "Leading Causes of Death," Centers for Disease Control and Prevention, last modified January 12, 2021, https://www.cdc.gov/nchs/fastats/leading-causes-of-death.htm.

14. "Limitations of Mammograms," American Cancer Society, last modified October 3, 2019, https://www.cancer.org/cancer/breast-cancer/screening-tests-and-early-detection/mammograms/limitations-of-mammograms.html.

15. Hui-Ling Chen et al., "A Support Vector Machine Classifier with Rough Set-Based Feature Selection for Breast Cancer Diagnosis," Expert Systems with Applications 38, no. 7 (2011): 9014–9022.

16. Chen et al., "A Support Vector," 9014.

17. D'Ignazio and Klein, Data, 28.

18. Lawrence, "Siri Disciplines," 179.

19. Judith S. Jacobson et al., "Breast Biopsy and Race/Ethnicity among Women without Breast Cancer," Cancer Detection and Prevention 30, no. 2 (2006): 129–133.

20. Jacobson et al., "Breast Biopsy," 131.

21. Chen et al., "A Support Vector," 9015.

22. Ibid., 9020.

23. A. Moran-Thomas, "Oximeters Used to Be Designed for Equity. What Happened?," Wired, June 4, 2021, https://www.wired.com/story/pulse-oximeters-equity/.

24. Gennatas and Chen, "Artificial," 7.

25. Tom M. Mitchell, "The Discipline of Machine Learning," 2006, http://www.cs.cmu.edu/~tom/pubs/MachineLearning.pdf, 1.

26. Computer scientists often have interesting ways of expressing themselves. Just to be clear, P is a variable like T (task) or E (experience) in Mitchell's definition. It's not a specific benchmarking metric. There's no formula for P. The Doctor and the Algorithm explores several specific metrics in Chapter 4.

27. Chen et al., "A Support Vector," 9015.

28. Ibid., 9019.

29. Ibid.

30. Latour, Science, 131.

CHAPTER 2

1. Hippocrates, *The Book of Prognostics*, Internet Classics Archive, accessed April 21, 2021, http://classics.mit.edu/Hippocrates/prognost.mb.txt.
2. John M. Thomas, Leo M. Cooney, and Terri R. Fried, "Prognosis Reconsidered in Light of Ancient Insights—from Hippocrates to Modern Medicine," *JAMA Internal Medicine 179*, no. 6 (2019): 820–823, 820.
3. Institute of Medicine (US) Committee for the Study of the Future of Public Health, *The Future of Public Health* (Washington, DC: National Academies Press [US], 1988), Chapter 3, A History of the Public Health System. Available from: https://www.ncbi.nlm.nih.gov/books/NBK218224.
4. World Health Organization, "Smallpox Vaccines," May 31, 2016, https://www.who.int/news-room/feature-stories/detail/smallpox-vaccines.
5. Myron Schultz, "Rudolf Virchow," *Emerging Infectious Diseases 14*, no. 9 (2008): 1480.
6. Graham, *Politics*, 141.
7. Andrew Whyte Barclay, *A Manual of Medical Diagnosis* (Philadelphia, PA: Blanchard & Lea, 1862), 29.
8. Thomas et al., "Prognosis Reconsidered," 820.
9. Jacob Yerushalmy, "Statistical Problems in Assessing Methods of Medical Diagnosis, with Special Reference to X-ray Techniques," Public Health Reports (1896–1970) (1947): 1432–1449.
10. Yerushalmy, "Statistical Problems," 1432.
11. See Chapter 4 for more details on the calculation of these metrics.
12. Graham, *Politics*, 44.
13. Thomas et al., "Prognosis Reconsidered," 820.
14. Topol, *Deep Medicine*, 186.
15. Santiago Romero-Brufau et al., "The Fifth Vital Sign? Nurse Worry Predicts Inpatient Deterioration within 24 hours," *JAMIA Open 2*, no. 4 (2019): 465–470.
16. Romero-Brufau, "The Fifth," 465.
17. Ibid.
18. Ibid., 466.
19. Ibid., 468.
20. Thomas et al., "Prognosis Reconsidered," 821.
21. Ibid.
22. Topol, *Deep Medicine*, 235.
23. M.J. Soares et al., "Conflict of Interest in Nutrition Research: An Editorial Perspective" *European Journal of Clinical Nutrition 73*, no. 9 (2019): 1213–1215.
24. Topol, *Deep Medicine*, 241.
25. Ibid., 242.
26. Ibid., 267.
27. David Zeevi et al., "Personalized Nutrition by Prediction of Glycemic Responses," *Cell 163*, no. 5 (2015): 1079–1094.
28. Ibid., 1081.
29. ,T.M.S. Wolever, "Personalized Nutrition by Prediction of Glycaemic Responses: Fact or Fantasy?" European Journal of Clinical Nutrition *70*, no. 4 (2016): 411–413.

30. Ibid., 411.

31. Ibid., 412.

32. Patrice D. Cani, "Human Gut Microbiome: Hopes, Threats and Promises," Gut 67, no. 9 (2018): 1716–1725, 1720.

33. Dina Hamideh et al., "Your Digital Nutritionist," The Lancet 393, no. 10166 (2019): 19.

34. See, for example, Simple Life, "Simple Fasting App Will provide Personalized Dieting Tips through AI-powered Functionality," Cision PR Newswire, February 4, 2020, https://www.prnewswire.com/news-releases/simple-fasting-app-will-provide-personalized-dieting-tips-through-ai-powered-functionality-300996 820.html.

35. Topol, Deep Medicine, 267.

36. M. Matheny, S. Thadaney Israni, and M. Ahmed, Artificial Intelligence in Health Care: The Hope, the Hype, the Promise, the Peril (National Academy of Medicine, 2020), 63.

37. Jaeho et al., "Roles of Artificial Intelligence in Wellness, Healthy Living, and Healthy Status Sensing, in Artificial Intelligence in Medicine, 151.

38. Ibid.

39. https://vesselhealth.com/.

40. Michael Marmot and Richard Wilkinson, eds., Social Determinants of Health (Oxford: OUP, 2005); WHO Commission on Social Determinants of Health, and World Health Organization, Closing the Gap in a Generation: Health Equity through Action on the Social Determinants of Health: Commission on Social Determinants of Health Final Report (Genevea: World Health Organization, 2008).

41. Baobao Zhang and Allan Dafoe, "Artificial Intelligence: American Attitudes and Trends," Available at SSRN 3312874 (2019). https://papers.ssrn.com/sol3/papers.cfm?abstract_id=3312874.

42. Zhang and Dafoe, "Artificial Intelligence."

43. Onur Asan, Alparslan Emrah Bayrak, and Avishek Choudhury, "Artificial Intelligence and Human Trust in Healthcare: Focus on Clinicians," Journal of Medical Internet Research 22, no. 6 (2020): e15154. https://www.jmir.org/2020/6/e15154/.

44. Forough Poursabzi-Sangdeh et al., "Manipulating and Measuring Model Interpretability," in CHI Conference on Human Factors in Computing Systems (CHI '21), May 8–13, 2021, Yokohama, Japan (New York: ACM, 2021), https://doi.org/10.1145/3411764.3445315.

45. Marzyeh Ghassemi et al., "Clinicalvis: Supporting Clinical Task-focused Design Evaluation," arXiv preprint arXiv:1810.05798 (2018). https://arxiv.org/abs/1810.05798; Gagan Bansal et al., "Does the Whole Exceed Its Parts? The Effect of AI Explanations on Complementary Team Performance," arXiv preprint arXiv:2006.14779 (2020), https://arxiv.org/abs/2006.14779.

46. Frank Pascale, New Laws of Robotics (Cambridge, MA: Harvard University Press, 2020).

47. Malin Eiband et al., "The Impact of Placebic Explanations on Trust in Intelligent Systems," in Extended Abstracts of the 2019 CHI Conference on Human Factors in

Computing Systems, 1–6 (2019); Zana Buçinca et al., "Proxy Tasks and Subjective Measures Can Be Misleading in Evaluating Explainable AI Systems," in *Proceedings of the 25th International Conference on Intelligent User Interfaces*, 454–464 (2020).

48. J.M. Heilman et al., 2011, Wikipedia: A Key Tool for Global Public Health Promotion, Journal of Medical Internet Research 13, *no.* 20111: e14. https://www.jmir.org/2011/1/e14/.
49. STAT, *Promise*, 159.
50. Broussard, *Artificial Unintelligence*, 7–8.
51. Ibid., 8.
52. Ibid.
53. Benjamin, *Race after*, 141.
54. O'Neil, *Weapons*, 25.
55. Noble, *Algorithms*, 2.
56. Berci Meskó, Twitter post, March 23, 2021, 10:00 a.m., https://twitter.com/Berci/status/1374375523082629143.
57. Topol, *Deep Medicine*, 204.
58. Ibid., 177.
59. Ibid., 164.
60. Ibid., 274.
61. Arjun Panesar, *Machine Learning and AI for Healthcare: Big Data for Improved Health Outcomes*, 2nd ed. (New York: Apress, 2021), 213.
62. Ibid., 212.
63. Ibid., 212–213.
64. Ibid., 223.
65. Ibid.
66. Ibid., 223–225.
67. Peter Micca et al., "Trends in Health Yech Investments: Funding the Future of Health," Deloitte Insights, February 26, 2021, https://www2.deloitte.com/us/en/insights/industry/health-care/health-tech-private-equity-venture-capital.html.
68. Melinda E. Cooper, Life as Surplus: Biotechnology and Capitalism in the Neoliberal Era (Seattle: University of Washington Press, 2011).
69. Cooper, *Life as Surplus*, 19.
70. Christa Teston, "Pathologizing Precarity," in Precarious Rhetorics, ed. Wendy S. Hesford, Adela C. Licona, and Christa Teston, 276–298 (Columbus: The Ohio State University Press, 2018).
71. Latour, *Science*, 137.

CHAPTER 3

1. Catherine Price, "The Age of Scurvy," Distillations 3, no. 2 (2018): 12–23.
2. Everett Rogers, Diffusion of Innovations (New York: Free Press, 2003).
3. James Lind, A Treatise on Scurvy in Three Parts (Edinburgh: Sands, Murray and Conchran, 1753).
4. Lind, *A Treatise*, 192.

5. James Lind, An Essay on the Most Effectual Means of Preserving the Health of Seamen, in the Royal Navy (London: A. Millar, 1757).

6. Gilbert Blane, *A Short Account of the Most Effectual Means of Preserving the Health of Seamen, Particularly in the Royal Navy* (London, 1780).

7. Vinay Prasad and Adam Cifu, "Medical Reversal: Why We Must Raise the Bar before Adopting New Technologies," Yale Journal of Biology and Medicine *84*, no. 4 (2011): 471–478.

8. Rebecca Y. Lin and Jeffery B. Alvarez, "Industry Perspectives and Commercial Opportunities of Artificial Intelligence in Medicine," in Artificial Intelligence in Medicine: Technical Basis and Clinical Applications, ed. Lei Xing, Maryellen L. Giger, and James K. Min (London: Academic Press, 2021), 492.

9. Joseph L. Bower and Clayton M. Christensen, "Disruptive Technologies: Catching the Wave," Harvard Business Review (1995), https://hbr.org/1995/01/disruptive-technologies-catching-the-wave.

10. Chris Velazco, "Facebook Can't Move Fast to Fix the Things It Broke," *Engaget*, April 12, 2018, https://www.engadget.com/2018-04-12-facebook-has-no-quick-solutions.html.

11. Meredith Broussard, Artificial Unintelligence: How Computers Misunderstand the World (Cambridge, MA: The MIT Press, 2019), 75.

12. Broussard, *Artificial*, 85.

13. Topol, *Deep Medicine*, 14.

14. Lin and Alverez, "Industry Perspectives," 492.

15. Ibid.

16. Ibid.

17. Donna J. Haraway's Modest Witness@Second_Millenium.FemaleMan©_Meets_On coMouse™: Feminism and Technoscience (New York and London: Routledge, 1997) offers a detailed analysis of the many ways science and marketing are interpenetrated in biomedical innovation.

18. Prasad and Cifu, "Medical Reversal," 471.

19. Vinayak K. Prasad and Adam S. Cifu, Ending Medical Reversal: Improving Outcomes, Saving Lives (Baltimore: Johns Hopkins University Press, 2015), 11.

20. Prasad and Cifu, *Ending Medical*, 17–18.

21. Albert L. Siu, "Screening for Breast Cancer: US Preventive Services Task Force Recommendation Statement," Annals of Internal Medicine *164*, no. 4 (2016): 279–296; Kevin C. Oeffinger et al., "Breast Cancer Screening for Women at Average Risk: 2015 Guideline Update from the American Cancer Society," JAMA *314*, no. 15 (2015): 1599–1614; Committee on Gynecologic Practice, "Committee Opinion No. 625: Management of Women with Dense Breasts Diagnosed by Mammography. American College of Obstetricians and Gynecologists," Obstetrics & Gynecology *125*, no. 3 (2015): 750–751; Beatrice Lauby-Secretan et al., "Breast-Cancer Screening—Viewpoint of the IARC Working Group," New England Journal of Medicine *372*, no. 24 (2015): 2353–2358; American Academy of Family Physicians, "Summary of Recommendations for Clinical Preventive Services." April 2016, http://www.aafp.org/dam/AAFP/documents/patient_care/clinical_recommendations/cps-recommendations.pdf.

22. Prasad and Cifu, *Ending Medical*, 277.
23. Kristin Compton, "Vioxx," DrugWatch, n.d., https://www.drugwatch.com/vioxx.
24. Prasad and Cifu, *Ending Medical*, 162.
25. Prasad and Cifu, "Medical Reversal," 474.
26. Although, they describe reversal as essentially inevitable, Prasad and Cifu offer a number of targeted recommendations designed to limit its occurrence. See *Ending Medical Reversal* for a full account.
27. Latour, *Science*, 137.
28. In the subsequent section, however, my exploration of toe fungus AI focuses on portability and dissemination in a more hopeful case of open science in action.
29. iCAD, "iCAD Announces FDA Clearance of ProFound AI™ for Digital Breast Tomosynthesis," December 7, 2018, https://www.icadmed.com/newsroom.html#!/posts/iCAD-Announces-FDA-Clearance-of-ProFound-AI-for-Digital-Breast-Tomosynthesis/124.
30. iCAD, Inc., "ProFound AI™ for 2D Mammography and Tomosynthesis,"n.d., https://pdf.medicalexpo.com/pdf/icad/profound-ai-2d-mammography-tomosynthesis/100519-212559.html.
31. FDA, "510(k) Clearances," September 2018, https://www.fda.gov/medical-devices/device-approvals-denials-and-clearances/510k-clearances.
32. iCAD, "Artificial Intelligence for Digital Breast Tomosynthesis - Reader Study Results." Revision B. white paper, 2020, https://www.icadmed.com/assets/dmm253-reader-studies-results-rev-b.pdf.
33. Broussard, *Artificial Unintelligence*, 175.
34. Topol, *Deep Medicine*, 18.
35. David Lyell et al., "How Machine Learning Is Embedded to Support Clinician Decision Making: An Analysis of FDA-approved Medical Devices," BMJ Health & Care Informatics *28*, no. 1 (2021): 1.
36. FDA, "Non-Inferiority Clinical Trials to Establish Effectiveness: Guidance for Industry," November 2016, https://www.fda.gov/media/78504/download.
37. Vinayak K. Prasad, Malignant: How Bad Policy and Bad Evidence Harm People with Cancer (Baltimore: Johns Hopkins University Press, 2020), 161.
38. iCAD, "Artificial Intelligence for Digital Breast Tomosynthesis - Reader Study Results." Revision A. white paper, 2018, https://www.icadmed.com/assets/dmm253-reader-studies-results-rev-a.pdf.
39. iCAD, "iCAD Unveils ProFound AI™ for Digital Breast Tomosynthesis at RSNA 2018," November 26, 2018, https://www.icadmed.com/newsroom.html#!/posts/iCAD-Unveils-ProFound-AI-for-Digital-Breast-Tomosynthesis-at-RSNA-2018/123.
40. FDA to iCAD Inc., December 6, 2018, https://www.accessdata.fda.gov/cdrh_docs/pdf18/K182373.pdf.
41. iCAD, "iCAD Announces FDA Clearance of ProFound AI™ for Digital Breast Tomosynthesis," December 7, 2018, https://www.icadmed.com/newsroom.html#!/posts/iCAD-Announces-FDA-Clearance-of-ProFound-AI-for-Digital-Breast-Tomosynthesis/124.

42. iCAD, "ProFound AI® for Digital Breast Tomosynthesis,"n.d., https://www.icad
    med.com/profoundai.html.

43. iCAD, "ProFound AI™ for Digital Breast Tomosynthesis,"n.d., https://www.icad
    med.com/assets/dmm252_profound_ai_for_breast_tomosynthesis_revb.pdf.

44. Benjamin, *Race after*, 30.

45. Emily F. Conant et al., "Improving Accuracy and Efficiency with Concurrent Use
    of Artificial Intelligence for Digital Breast Tomosynthesis," Radiology-Artificial
    Intelligence *1*, no. 4, e180096. https://pubs.rsna.org/doi/full/10.1148/ryai.201
    9180096.

46. Emily F. Conant et al., "Association of Digital Breast Tomosynthesis vs Digital
    Mammography with Cancer Detection and Recall Rates by Age and Breast
    Density," JAMA Oncology 5, no. 5 (2019): 635–642.

47. In this industry marketing context, it is important to remember the double-edged
    sword of inclusion. As Benjamin notes, diverse inclusion in clinical trials is often a
    proxy for market penetration, "a lucrative stand-in for social and political justice;"
    Race after, 157.

48. Radiology Society of North America (RSNA), "RSNA 2020 Booth Space Selection
    Guidelines,"n.d., https://www.rsna.org/-/media/Files/RSNA/Annual-meeting/Exh
    ibitors/Tools-and-guides/2020-booth-space-selection-guidelines_final.ashx.

49. The ICE Community, https://theicecommunity.com/.

50. "iCAD Reports over 1,000 Licenses Sold as Part of ProFound AI Sales," *ICE
    Magazine*, November 24, 2020, https://theicecommunity.com/icad-reports-over-
    1000-licenses-sold-as-part-of-profound-ai-sales/.

51. iCAD, "iCAD Reports over 1,000 Licenses Sold as Part of ProFound AI Sales,"
    November 24, 2020, https://www.icadmed.com/newsroom.html#!/posts/iCAD-
    Reports-Over-1000-Licenses-Sold-as-Part-of-ProFound-AI-Sales/232.

52. Nancy Pontika et al., "Fostering Open Science to Research using a Taxonomy and
    an eLearning Portal" (paper presented at iKnow: 15th International Conference on
    Knowledge Technologies and Data Driven Business, Graz, Austria, October 21–
    22, 2015).

53. FOSTER, "What Is Open Science? Introduction," n.d., https://www.fosteropenscie
    nce.eu/content/what-open-science-introduction.

54. Joseph M. Gabriel, Medical Monopoly: Intellectual Property Rights and the
    Origin of the Modern Pharmaceutical Industry (Chicago: University of Chicago
    Press, 2014).

55. Seung Seog Han et al., "Deep Neural Networks Show an Equivalent and Often
    Superior Performance to Dermatologists in Onychomycosis Diagnosis: Automatic
    Construction of Onychomycosis Datasets by Region-Based Convolutional Deep
    Neural Network," Plos-One *13*, no. 1, e0191493. https://doi.org/10.1371/journal.
    pone.0191493.

56. Ibid., 17.

57. See the Hal et al. article for a very graphic illustration of this process.

58. Han et al., "Deep Neural," 2.

59. Ibid., 5.

60. Ibid., 15.

61. Yin Yang et al., "Development and Validation of Two Artificial Intelligence Models for Diagnosing Benign, Pigmented Facial Skin Lesions," Skin Research and Technology, August 8, 2020, https://doi.org/10.1111/srt.12911.

62. Ursula Schmidt-Erfurth et al., "Artificial Intelligence in Retina," *Progress in Retinal and Eye Research 67* (2018): 1–29.

63. S.I. Cho et al., "Dermatologist-Level Classification of Malignant Lip Diseases Using a Deep Convolutional Neural Network," British Journal of Dermatology *182*, no. 6 (2020): 1388–1394.

64. Benjamin, *Race after*, 59.

65. Preetha Kamath et al., "Visual Racism in Internet Searches and Dermatology Textbooks," Journal of the American Academy of Dermatology, October 2020, https://www.sciencedirect.com/science/article/pii/S0190962220328930; Robert J. Smith and Brittany U. Oliver, "Advocating for Black Lives—a Call to Dermatologists to Dismantle Institutionalized Racism and Address Racial Health Inequities," JAMA Dermatology, November 25, 2020, https://jamanetwork.com/journals/jama dermatology/article-abstract/2773122.

CHAPTER 4

1. Jeremy Laurance, "The Doctors Had Given Up. They Said Her Heart Had Stopped and She Had Brain Damage. But She's Fine," The Independent, October 15, 2012, https://www.independent.co.uk/life-style/health-and-families/health-news/doct ors-had-given-they-said-her-heart-had-stopped-and-she-had-brain-damage-she-s-fine-8211015.html.

2. Harmmet Kaur, "Family of Woman Who Died Weeks after She Was Found Alive at a Funeral Home Sues Paramedics for $50 Million," CNN Online, October 20, 2020 https://www.cnn.com/2020/10/20/us/timesha-beauchamp-dies-lawsuit-trnd/index.html.

3. Vedamurthy Adhiyaman, Sonja Adhiyaman, and Radha Sundaram, "The Lazarus Phenomenon," Journal of the Royal Society of Medicine *100*, no. 12 (2007): 552–557.

4. Jérémie F. Cohen et al., "Rapid Antigen Detection Tests for Group A Streptococcus in Children with Pharyngitis," *Cochrane Database of Systematic Reviews*, no. 7 (2016), CD010502. DOI: 10.1002/14651858.CD010502.pub2.

5. And Avanti et al., "Improving Palliative Care with Deep Learning," arXiv (2017), https://arxiv.org/pdf/1711.06402.pdf.

6. Laurence O'Dwyer et al., "Using Support Vector Machines with Multiple Indices of Diffusion for Automated Classification of Mild Cognitive Impairment," Plos-One7, no. 2 (2012): e32441. https://doi.org/10.1371/journal.pone.0032441.

7. Jordyn Phelps, "Trump Keeps Bragging about Acing Simple Test Used to Detect Mental Impairment," ABC News, July 23, 2020, https://abcnews.go.com/Politics/trump-bragging-acing-simple-test-detect-mental-impairment/story?id=71945342.

8. Mini-Mental State Exam (MMSE), retrieved February 2021, https://www.ncbi.nlm.nih.gov/projects/gap/cgi-bin/GetPdf.cgi?id=phd001525.1.

9. Alex J. Mitchell, "A Meta-Analysis of the Accuracy of the Mini-mental State Examination in the Detection of Dementia and Mild Cognitive Impairment," Journal of Psychiatric Research 43, no. 4 (2008): 411–431.

10. Erping Long et al., "An Artificial Intelligence Platform for the Multihospital Collaborate Management of Congenital Cataracts," Nature Biomedical Engineering 1 (2017): 0024. https://www.nature.com/articles/s41551-016-0024.

11. Juan J. Gómez-Valverde et al., "Automatic Glaucoma Classification Using Color Fundus Images Based on Convolutional Neural Networks and Transfer Learning," Biomedical Optics Express 10, no. 2 (2019): 892–913.

12. Rory Sayres et al., "Using a Deep Learning Algorithm and Integrated Gradients Explanation to Assist Grading for Diabetic Retinopathy," Ophthalmology 126, no. 4 (2019): 552–564. https://doi.org/10.1016/j.ophtha.2018.11.016.

13. Lachlan J. Gunn et al., "Too Good to Be True: When Overwhelming Evidence Fails to Convince," Proceedings of the Royal Society A 472, no. 2187 (2016): 20150748.

14. Chao Zhang et al., "Toward an Expert Level of Lung Cancer Detection and Classification Using a Deep Convolutional Neural Network," The Oncologist 24, no. 9 (2019): 1159–1165.

15. Lisa Zyga, "Why Too Much Evidence Can Be a Bad Thing," Phys.org, January 4, 2016, https://phys.org/news/2016-01-evidence-bad.html.

16. Anton S. Becker et al., "Classification of Breast Cancer in Ultrasound Imaging Using a Generic Deep Learning Analysis Software: A Pilot Study," British Journal of Radiology 91 (2018): 1083.

17. These are often called "reliability" and "validity," but I'm going to use the terms that are more common in health AI.

18. This is a made-up number. As best I can tell, Gmail doesn't report its spam detection AUC score, but it does brag about an accuracy [TP + TN/(TP + FP + TN + FN)] of 99.9%. See Cade Metz, "Google Says Its AI Catches 99.9 Percent of Gmail Spam," Wired, July 9, 2015, https://www.wired.com/2015/07/google-says-ai-catches-99-9-percent-gmail-spam/.

19. Terry K. Koo and Mae Y. Li, "A Guideline of Selecting and Reporting Intraclass Correlation Coefficients for Reliability Research," Journal of Chiropractic Medicine 15, no. 2 (2016): 155–163.

20. Domenic Vincent Cicchetti, "Guidelines, Criteria, and Rules of Thumb for Evaluating Normed and Standardized Assessment Instruments in Psychology, Psychological Assessment 6, no. 4 (1994): 284.

21. Joseph L. Fleiss, Design and Analysis of Clinical Experiments (New York: John Wiley & Sons, 2011).

22. Food and Drug Administration, Guidance for Industry and FDA Staff: Statistical Guidance on Reporting Results from Studies Evaluating Diagnostic Tests, March 13, 2007, https://www.fda.gov/media/71147/download, 17.

23. Arie Ben-David, "About the Relationship between ROC Curves and Cohen's Kappa," Engineering Applications of Artificial Intelligence 21, no. 6 (2008): 874–882.

24. "William F. Baker (engineer)," Wikipedia, accessed February 28, 2021, https://en.wikipedia.org/wiki/William_F._Baker_(engineer).

25. Andrew Bloom, "Engineer Bill Baker Is the King of Superstable 150-Story Structures," Wired, November 27, 2007, https://www.wired.com/2007/11/mf-baker/.
26. Additional details about the data set and simulation methodology are available in the Technical Appendix (sections A.1.1–A.1.3).
27. See Chapter 1 for a more detailed discussion of this data set.
28. Additional details about this simulation are described in section 1.4 of the Technical Appendix.
29. Agreement metrics are highly interoperable and often identical to several significant digits when used to evaluate the same confusion matrix. Nevertheless, we can be confident that CCC = 0.35 is well below κ = 0.75.
30. Hyunkwant Lee et al., "An Explainable Deep-Learning Algorithm for the Detection of Acute Intracranial Haemorrhage from Small Datasets," Nature Biomedical Engineering 3, no. 3 (2019), 173–182.
31. Ibid., 174.
32. Ibid., 177.
33. Ibid.
34. Andrew Wong et al., "External Validation of a Widely Implemented Proprietary Sepsis Prediction Model in Hospitalized Patients," JAMA Internal Medicine 181, no. 8 (2021): 1065–1070.
35. Ibid., 1067.
36. Xiaoxuan Liu et al., "A Comparison of Deep Learning Performance against Health-Care Professionals in Detecting Diseases from Medical Imaging: A Systematic Review and Meta-Analysis," The Lancet Digital Health 1, no. 6 (2019): e271–e297.
37. Ibid., e271.
38. One study used an external validity assessment but also trained the AI based on a non-reference standard. This study is not included in the count of platinum standard studies since both use of the reference standard and external validity are required to reach the platinum standard.
39. Liu et al., "A Comparison," e271.

CHAPTER 5

1. Matheny et al., "Artificial Intelligence," 16.
2. Ibid., 91.
3. Ibid., 91.
4. Stephen Hilgartner, "The Dominant View of Popularization: Conceptual Problems, Political Uses," Social Studies of Science 20, no. 3 (1990): 519–539; 519.
5. Yingya Li, Jieke Zhang, and Bei Yu, "An NLP Analysis of Exaggerated Claims in Science News," in Proceedings of the 2017 EMNLP Workshop: Natural Language Processing Meets Journalism (Copenhagen: Association for Computational Linguistics, 2017): 106–111.
6. Jasabanta Patro and Sabyasachee Baruah, "A Simple Three-Step Approach for the Automatic Detection of Exaggerated Statements in Health Science News," in Proceedings of the 16th Conference of the European Chapter of the Association

for Computational Linguistics: Main Volume (Association for Computational Linguistics, 2021), 3293–3305.

7. Bei Yu et al., "Measuring Correlation-to-Causation Exaggeration in Press Releases," in Proceedings of the 28th International Conference on Computational Linguistics (Barcelona: International Committee on Computational Linguistics, 2020), 4860–4872.

8. Kevin Lomangino, "It's Time for AAAS and EurekAlert! to Crack Down on Misinformation in PR News Releases," Health News Review, October 2018, https://www.healthnewsreview.org/2018/10/its-time-for-aaas-and-eurekalert-to-crack-down-on-misinformation-in-pr-news-releases/.

9. Northwestern University, "AI Tools Speeds Up Search for COVID-19 Treatments and Vaccines," EurekAlert!, May 4, 2020, https://www.eurekalert.org/pub_releases/2020-05/nu-ats042920.php.

10. Babylon, "AI with 'Imagination' Could Help Doctors with Diagnosis, Particularly for Complex Case," EurekAlert!, August 11, 2020, https://www.eurekalert.org/pub_releases/2020-08/b-aw081020.php.

11. Binghamton University, "Big Data-Driven Method Could Save Money, Increase Efficiency in Pharmaceutical Management," EurekAlert!, March 29, 2016, https://www.eurekalert.org/pub_releases/2016-03/bu-bdm032916.php.

12. Ibid.

13. eLife, "New AI Tool Speeds Up Biology and Removes Potential Human Bias," EurekAlert!, November 3, 2020, https://www.eurekalert.org/pub_releases/2020-11/e-natl10320.php.

14. John Lynch et al., "Bridging Science and Journalism: Identifying the Role of Public Relations in the Construction and Circulation of Stem Cell Research among Laypeople," *Science Communication 36*, no. 4 (2014): 479–501.

15. Ibid., 483.

16. Ibid.

17. *Narrator*: They do not.

18. Chiara Longoni and Carey K. Morewedge, "AI Can Outperform Doctors. So Why Don't Patients Trust It?," Harvard Business Review, October 30, 2019, https://hbr.org/2019/10/ai-can-outperform-doctors-so-why-dont-patients-trust-it.

19. Zachary Hendrickson, "Google's DeepMind AI Outperforms Doctors in Identifying Breast Cancer from X-Ray Images," Business Insider, January 3, 2020, https://www.businessinsider.com/google-deepmind-outperforms-doctors-identifying-breast-cancer-2020-1.

20. Denise Grady, "A.I. Took a Test to Detect Lung Cancer. It got an A," The New York Times, May 20, 2019, https://www.nytimes.com/2019/05/20/health/cancer-artific ial-intelligence-ct-scans.html.

21. Ruth Reader, "Why Google, Amazon, and Nvidia Are All Building AI Notetakers for Doctors," November 13, 2020, https://www.fastcompany.com/90555218/google-amazon-nvidia-ai-medical-transcription.

22. Lynch et al., "Bridging Science," 491–492.

23. Fergus Walsh, "AI 'Outpreforms' Doctors Diagnosing Breast Cancer," BBC News, January 2, 2020, https://www.bbc.com/news/health-50857759.

24. Scott Mayer McKinney et al., "International Evaluation of an AI System for Breast Cancer Screening," Nature 577 (2020): 89–94, 89.

25. Ryan O'Hare, "Artificial Intelligence Could Help to Spot Breast Cancer," *Imperial College London news site*, January 2020, https://www.imperial.ac.uk/news/194506/artificial-intelligence-could-help-spot-breast/.

26. Anton S. Becker et al., "Classification of Breast Cancer in Ultrasound Imaging Using a Generic Deep Learning Analysis Software: A Pilot Study," British Journal of Radiology 91 (2018): 2017056, https://doi.org/10.1259/bjr.20170576, 1.

27. Seung Seog Han et al., "Deep Neural Networks Show an Equivalent and Often Superior Performance to Dermatologists in Onychomycosis Diagnosis: Automatic Construction of Onychomycosis Datasets by Region-based Convolutional Deep Neural Network," *Plos-One 13*, no. 1 (2018): e019493, https://doi.org/10.1371/journal.pone.0191493, 12.

28. James M. Brown et al., "Automated Diagnosis of Plus Disease in Retinopathy of Prematurity Using Deep Convolutional Neural Networks," JAMA Ophthalmology 136, no. 7 (2018): 803–810, 807.

29. Haraway, *Modest.Witness*, 197.

30. Ibid., 199.

31. D'Ignazio and Klein, *Data Feminism*, 17.

32. Ibid., 35.

33. Liu et al., "A Comparison."

34. S. Scott Graham and Hannah R. Hopkins, "AI for Social Justice: New Methodological Horizons in Technical Communication." *Technical Communication Quarterly 31*, no. 1 (2021): 89–102.

35. More complete details on how POS aveloc works and subsequent modeling are available in the Technical Appendix (sections A.2.2 and A.2.3, respectively).

36. John M. Swales and Christine B. Feak, Academic Writing for Graduate Students: Essential Tasks and Skills. Vol. 1 (Ann Arbor: University of Michigan Press, 2004).

37. Li Zhou and Margarita Sordo, "Expert Systems in Medicine," in *Artificial Intelligence in Medicine*, 76.

38. Karen Drukker et al., "Biomedical Imaging and Analysis through Deep Learning," in Artificial Intelligence in Medicine, 63.

39. Spearman's ρ = .0821, p = 0447. Further details on all statistical tests performed in this chapter can be found in section A.2.4 of the Technical Appendix.

40. χ^2 = 3.9, p = 0.0483.

41. 95% CI: 0.0371–0.0898.

42. Jakob D. Jensen, "Scientific Uncertainty in News Coverage of Cancer Research: Effects of Hedging on Scientists' and Journalists' Credibility," Human Communication Research 34, no. 3 (2008): 347–369.

43. Ryan Omizo and William Hart-Davidson, "Hedge-o-matic," enculturation 7 (2016), http://hedgeomatic.cal.msu.edu/hedgeomatic/.

44. Gavan J. Fitzsimons and Donald R. Lehmann, "Reactance to Recommendations: When Unsolicited Advice Yields Contrary Responses," Marketing Science 23, no. 1 (2004): 82–94.

45. Sections A.2.1–A.2.3 of the Technical Appendix provide further details on HedgeDx annotation, feature engineering, and model architecture.
46. Spearman's $\rho = 0.2043$, $p < 0.0001$.
47. Liu et al., "A Comparison," e271.

CHAPTER 6

1. Graham, *Politics*, 107.
2. Ibid., 121.
3. Ibid., 4–5.
4. Sascha Gruss et al., "Pain Intensity Recognition Rates via Biopotential Feature Patterns with Support Vector Machines," Plos One (2015), https://doi.org/10.1371/journal.pone.0140330.
5. Emma Pierson et al., "An Algorithm Approach to Reducing Unexplained Pain Disparities in Underserved Populations," Nature Medicine *27* (2021): 136–140.
6. O'Neil, *Weapons*, 204.
7. Andrew Burt, "Ethical Frameworks for AI Aren't Enough," Harvard Business Review, November 9, 2020, https://hbr.org/2020/11/ethical-frameworks-for-ai-arent-enough.
8. Melissa D. McCradden et al., "Ethical Limitations of Algorithmic Fairness Solutions in Health Care Machine Learning," The Lancet Digital Health *2*, no. 5 (2020): E221–E223; Alex John London, "Medical Decisions: Accuracy versus Explainability," Hastings Center Report *49*, no. 1 (2019): 15–21.
9. O'Neil, *Weapons*, 223.
10. Benjamin, *Race after*, 186.
11. Inioluwa Deborah Raji et al., "Closing the AI Accountability Gap: Defining an End-to-End Framework for Internal Algorithmic Auditing," in *Proceedings of the 2020 Conference on Fairness, Accountability, and Transparency*, (New York: Association for Computing Machinery, 2020), 33–44.
12. Benjamin, *Race after*, 186.
13. Robyn Caplan et al., Algorithmic Accountability: A Primer, Data & Society, 2019, https://datasociety.net/wp-content/uploads/2019/09/DandS_Algorithmic_Accountability.pdf.
14. Mullaney, "Your Computer," 6.
15. Kvita Philip, "How to Stop Worrying about Clean Signals," in Your Computer Is on Fire, ed. Thomas Mullaney et al. (Cambridge, MA: The MIT Press, 2021), 368–369.
16. See, for example, Denise Garcia, "Lethal Artificial Intelligence and Change: The Future of International Peace and Security," International Studies Review *20*, no. 2 (2018): 334–341.
17. Richard Drew, "IBM Abandons Facial Recognition Products, Condemns Racially Biased Surveillance," *NPR*, June 9, 2020, https://www.npr.org/2020/06/09/873298837/ibm-abandons-facial-recognition-products-condemns-racially-biased-surveillance.
18. Isobel Asher Hamilton, "Microsoft Took an Ethical Stand on Facial Recognition Just Days after Being Blasted for a Sinister AI Project in China," Business Insider,

      April 17, 2019, https://www.businessinsider.com/microsoft-refuses-to-sell-facial-
      recognition-tech-to-us-police-force-2019-4.
19.   Emily M. Bender et al., "On the Dangers of Stochastic Parrots: Can Language
      Models Be Too Big?," FAccT, 2021, https://faculty.washington.edu/ebender/papers/
      Stochastic_Parrots.pdf. This paper, of course, led to the forcible "resignating" of
      Timnit Gebru and Margaret Mitchell from their roles in Google's ethical AI di-
      vision. The resulting fallout has done much to showcase the severe limitations of
      in-house approaches to Ethical AI.
20.   Farah Master, "Computing Industry CO2 Emissions in the Spotlight," Reuters,
      January 15, 2009, https://www.reuters.com/article/us-computing-carbon-emissi
      ons/computing-industry-co2-emissions-in-the-spotlight-idUSTRE50E5QO2
      0090115.
21.   Adam R.H. Stevens et al., "The Imperative to Reduce Carbon Emissions in
      Astronomy," Nature Astronomy 4 (2020): 843–851.
22.   Bender et al., "On the Dangers," 3–4.
23.   Ibid., 2.
24.   A notable exception is Frank Pascale's New Laws of Robotics (Cambridge,
      MA: Harvard University Press, 2020), the second chapter of which focuses on legal
      and regulatory interventions to address the risks of ill-considered health AI (about
      which more will be presented in the next chapter).
25.   McCradden et al., "Ethical Limitations"; Frank Pasquale, New Laws of Robotics
      (Cambridge, MA: Harvard University Press, 2020).
26.   Alex John London, "Medical Decisions: Accuracy versus Explainability," Hastings
      Center Report 49, no. 1 (2019): 15–21.
27.   London, "Artificial Intelligence," 15.
28.   Ibid., 20.
29.   Philip, "How to Stop Worrying," 374.
30.   See, for example, Shane Neilson, "Ableism in the Medical Profession," Canadian
      Association Medical Journal 192, no. 15 (2020): e411–e412; Heidi L. Janz,
      "Ableism: The Undiagnosed Malady Afflicting Medicine," Canadian Association
      Medical Journal 191, no. 17 (2019): e478–e479; Joel Michael Reynolds, "Three
      Things Clinicians Should Know about Disability," AMA Journal of Ethics 20, no.
      12, e1181–e1187; Hannah Borowsky, Leonra Morinis, and Megha Garg, "Disability
      and Ableism in Medicine: A Curriculum for Medical Students," MedEd PORTAL
      17, no. 1 (2021): 11073.
31.   Joseph Shapiro, "People with Disabilities Fear Pandemic Will Worsen Medical
      Biases," NPR, April 15, 2020, https://www.npr.org/2020/04/15/828906002/people-
      with-disabilities-fear-pandemic-will-worsen-medical-biases; K. Herr et al., "Pain
      Assessment in the Nonverbal Patient: Position Statement with Clinical Practice
      Recommendations," Pain Management Nursing 7, no. 2 (2006): 44–52.
32.   Ibid.
33.   Gruss, Pain Intensity, 1.
34.   Ibid.
35.   Graham, Politics, 99.

36. K.J.S. Anand, "Re: Reply to Letters to the Editor from Merskey & Wall," PAIN 66, no. 1 (1996): 210.

37. Murat Aydede, "Does the IASP Definition of Pain Need Updating?," PAIN Reports 4, no. 5 (2019): e777.

38. Graham, *Politics*, 98–99.

39. Srinivasa Raja et al., "The Revised International Association for the Study of Pain Definition of Pain: Concepts, Challenges, and Compromises," PAIN 161, no. 9 (2020): 1976–1982.

40. "Nociception" is the technical term for the neural transmission of pain stimuli when pain is caused by a specific physical stimulus.

41. Sam Corbett-Davies and Sharad Goel, "The Measure and Mismeasure of Fairness: A Critical Review of Fair Machine Learning," arXiv preprint arXiv:1808.00023 (2018) https://arxiv.org/abs/1808.00023.

42. IBM, "AI Fairness 360," accessed April 8, 2021, https://aif360.mybluemix.net; Dave Gershgorn, "Facebook Says It Has a Tool to Detect Bias in Its Artificial Intelligence," Quartz, May 3, 2018, https://qz.com/1268520/facebook-says-it-has-a-tool-to-det ect-bias-in-its-artificial-intelligence/; Google, ML Fairness Gym, accessed April 8, 2021, https://github.com/google/ml-fairness-gym.

43. Kelly M. Hoffman et al., "Racial Bias in Pain Assessment and Treatment Recommendations, and False Beliefs about Biological Differences between Blacks and Whites," PNAS 113, no. 16 (2016): 4296–4301.

44. Lisa J. Stanton et al., "When Race Matters: Disagreements in Pain Perception between Patients and Their Physicians in Primary Care, *Journal of the National Medical Association* 99, no. 5 (2007): 532–838.

45. Kelly M. Hoffman et al., "Racial Bias."

46. Janice A. Sabin, "How We Fail Black Patients in Pain," Association of American Medical Colleges, January 6, 2020, https://www.aamc.org/news-insights/how-we-fail-black-patients-pain.

47. Pierson et al., "Algorithmic Approach," 136–140.

48. Ibid., 137.

49. J.H. Kellgren and Lawrence, "Radiological Assessment of Osteo-Arthrosis," Annals of the Rheumatic Diseases 16, no. 4 (1957): 494.

50. Karen Hao, "AI Could Make Health Care Fairer—by Helping Us Believe What Patients Say," MIT Technology Review, January 22, 2021, https://www.technolog yreview.com/2021/01/22/1016577/ai-fairer-healthcare-patient-outcomes/.

51. Pierson et al., "Algorithmic Approach," 139.

52. Hao, "AI Could Make."

53. Anne Underwood, "Next Frontiers: Fibromyalgia: Not All in Your Head," Newsweek, *May 19*, 2003, 53.

54. Catherine Poslusny, "How Much Does a PET Scan Cost?," New Choice Health, accessed April 8, 2021, https://www.newchoicehealth.com/pet-scan/cost.

55. See, for example, Ruha Benjamin, "Informed Refusal: Toward a Justice-Based Bioethics," Science, Technology, and Human Values 43, no. 6 (2016): 967–990.

56. Ruha Benjamin, "Assessing Risk, Automating Racism," *Science 366*, no. 6464 (2019): 421–422.

57. McCradden et al., "Ethical Limitations," e211.

58. Ibid.

59. American Medical Association, "Chapter 8: Opinions on Physicians & The Heath of the Community," AMA Principles of Medical Ethics, 2001, https://www.ama-assn.org/system/files/2020-12/code-of-medical-ethics-chapter-8.pdf.

60. Recently after a series of very public missteps, the AMA released an 83-page strategic plan promising a "pivot from ambivalence to urgent action" regarding racism in the organization. The plan does not outline any specific changes for the Code of Ethics; AMA, *Organizational Strategic Plan to Embed Racial Justice and Advance Health Equity 2021–2023*, 2021, https://www.ama-assn.org/system/files/2021-05/ama-equity-strategic-plan.pdf.

61. Daniel S. Goldberg, "Social Justice, Health Inequalities and Methodological Individualism in US Health Promotion," Public Health Ethics 5, no. 2 (2012): 104–115.

62. Rachel Fabi and Daniel S. Goldberg, "Bioethics, (Funding) Priorities, and the Perpetuation of Injustice," The American Journal of Bioethics (2021), https://doi.org/10.1080/15265161.2020.1867934.

63. McCradden et al., "Ethical Limitations," e222.

64. Chad Cook and Charles Sheets, "Clinical Equipoise and Personal Equipoise: Two Necessary Ingredients for Reducing Bias in Manual Therapy Trials," Journal of Manual & Manipulative Therapy 19, no. 1 (2011): 55–57.

CHAPTER 7

1. Google, *Perspectives on Issues in AI Governance*, accessed April 9, 2021, https://ai.google/static/documents/perspectives-on-issues-in-ai-governance.pdf, 2.

2. Benjamin, *Race after*, 186.

3. Noble, *Algorithms*, 133.

4. Hicks, "When Did the fire start?," in *Your Computer is on Fire*, ed. Thomas S. Mullaney, Benjamin Peters, Mar Hicks, and Kavita Philip, (Cambridge, MA: The MIT Press, 2021), 23.

5. Andrew Tutt, "An FDA for Algorithms," Administrative Law Review 69 (2017): 83.

6. United Nations, "Urgent Action Needed over Artificial intelligence Risks to Human Rights," UN News, September 15, 2021, https://news.un.org/en/story/2021/09/1099972.

7. AI Now Institute, "Algorithmic Accountability for the Public Sector: Learning from the First Wave of Policy Implementation," Medium, March 24, 2021, https://medium.com/@AINowInstitute/how-can-governments-keep-algorithms-accountable-a-look-at-the-first-wave-of-policy-implementation-312f4549469b.

8. See, for example, Melissa D. McCradden, Elizabeth A. Stephenson, and James A. Anderson, "Clinical Research Underlies Ethical Integration of Healthcare Artificial Intelligence," Nature Medicine 26, no. 9 (2020): 1325–1326; and Xiaoxuan Liu et al., "Reporting Guidelines for Clinical Trial Reports for Interventions Involving Artificial Intelligence: The CONSORT-AI Extension," bmj 370 (2020): m3164.

9. FDA, "Proposed Regulatory Framework for Modifications to Artificial Intelligence/Machine Learning (AI/ML)-B ased Software as a Medical Device

(SaMD): Discussion Paper and Request for Feedback," accessed April 9, 2021, https://www.fda.gov/files/medical%20devices/published/US-FDA-Artificial-Intelligence-and-Machine-Learning-Discussion-Paper.pdf.

10. Allan Dafoe, *AI Governance: A Research Agenda* (Oxford, UK: Centre for the Governance of AI, 2018), https://www.fhi.ox.ac.uk/wp-content/uploads/GovAI-Agenda.pdf.

11. Ayanna Howard, Jason Borenstein, and Kinnis Gosha, 2019, *NSF-Funded Fairness, Ethics, Accountability, and Transparency (FEAT) Workshop Report*, https://par.nsf.gov/servlets/purl/10139705.

12. D. Leslie et al., 2021, Artificial Intelligence, Human Rights, Democracy, and the Rule of Law: A Primer (The Council of Europe, 2021): https://rm.coe.int/primer-en-new-cover-pages-coe-english-compressed-2754-7186-0228-v-1/1680a2fd4a.

13. AI4People, "On Good AI Governance: 14 Priority Actions, a SMART Model of Governance, and a Regulatory Toolbox," November 7, 2019, https://ssrn.com/abstract=3486508.

14. European Commission, "On Artificial Intelligence—a European Approach to Excellence and Trust," 2018. https://ec.europa.eu/info/publications/white-paper-artificial-intelligence-european-approach-excellence-and-trust_en.

15. Elisa Jillson, "Aiming for Truth, Fairness, and Equity in Your Company's Use of AI," FTC, April 19, 2021, https://www.ftc.gov/news-events/blogs/business-blog/2021/04/aiming-truth-fairness-equity-your-companys-use-ai.

16. Dafoe, *AI Governance*, 28.

17. European Commission, "On Artificial," 10.

18. Poursabzi-Sangdeh et al., "Manipulating and Measuring Model Interpretability."

19. Jillson, "Aiming for Truth."

20. Leslie et al., *Artificial Intelligence*, 17.

21. Dafoe, *AI Governance*, 28.

22. Leslie et al., *Artificial Intelligence*, 5.

23. Caplan et al., *Algorithmic Accountability*, 4.

24. Jillson, "Aiming for Truth."

25. O'Neil, *Weapons*, 225.

26. European Commission, "On Artificial," 25.

27. Ibid.

28. Howard et al., *NSF-Funded*, 13.

29. D'Ignazio and Klein, *Data Feminism*, 65.

30. AI4People, "On Good AI," 18.

31. European Commission, "On Artificial," 25.

32. See, for example, Gene Rowe, and Lynn J. Frewer, "A Typology of Public Engagement Mechanisms," Science, Technology, & Human Values *30*, no. 2 (2005): 251–290; Michel Callon, Pierre Lascoumes, and Yannick Barthe, Acting in an Uncertain World: An Essay on Technical Democracy (Cambridge, MA: The MIT Press, 2011); Danielle DeVasto, Being Expert: L'Aquila and Issues of Inclusion in Science-Policy Decision Making, Social Epistemology 30, *no.* 4 (2016): 372–397; and Daniel J. Card, "Off-Target Impacts: Tracing Public Participation in Policy Making for

Agricultural Biotechnology," Journal of Business and Technical Communication *34*, no. 1 (2020): 77–103.

33. Caplan et al., *Algorithmic Accountability*, 25.
34. Leslie et al., *Artificial Intelligence*, 31.
35. Tutt, "An FDA," 111.
36. Ibid.
37. Ibid., 122.
38. See for example, Marcia Angell, The Truth about the Drug Companies: How They Deceive Us and What to Do about It (New York: Random House Incorporated, 2005); Carl Elliott, *White Coat, Black Hat: Adventures on the Dark Side of Medicine* (Boston: Beacon Press, 2010); Vinayak K. Prasad, Malignant: How Bad Policy and Bad Evidence Harm People with Cancer (Baltimore: JHU Press, 2020).
39. European Commission, "On Artificial," 8.
40. Leslie et al., *Artificial Intelligence*, 32.
41. Google, *Perspectives*, 28.
42. Howard et al., *NSF-Funded*, 16.
43. John A. Lynch, The Origins of Bioethics: Remembering When Medicine Went Wrong (East Lansing: MSU Press, 2019).
44. 21 U.S. Code § 679—Application of Federal Food, Drug, and Cosmetic Act.
45. WHO Scientific Group, *Guidelines for Evaluation of Drugs for Use in Man*. (Geneva: World Health Organization, 1975), 10.
46. WHO, *Ethics and Governance of Artificial Intelligence for Health: WHO Guidance* (Geneva: World Health Organization, 2021).
47. Pascale, *New Laws*, 44–48.
48. McCraddon et al., "Clinical Research," 1325.
49. Eric Wu et al., "How Medical AI Devices Are Evaluated: Limitations and Recommendations from an Analysis of FDA Approvals," Nature Medicine 57 (2021): 582–584.
50. McCraddon et al., "Clinical Research," 1325.
51. Wu et al., "How Medical," 2.
52. FDA, "Proposed Regulatory," 9.
53. Eric J. Topol, "Welcoming New Guidelines for AI Clinical Research," Nature Medicine *26*, no. 9 (2020): 1318–1320; 1319.
54. STAT, *Promise and Peril: How Artificial Intelligence Is Transforming Healthcare*, 2021, https://www.statnews.com/wp-content/uploads/2021/04/STAT_Promise_an d_Peril_2021_Report.pdf, 13.
55. Topol, "Welcoming," 1318.
56. Ivan Oransky, "NIH Suspended Some Grants to Duke amid Concern for Patient Safety," *Medscape*, May 21, 2019, https://www.medscape.com/viewarticle/913283.
57. Elliott, *White Coat*.
58. FDA, "Proposed Regulatory," 8.
59. Eric Wu et al., "How Medical," 27: 584.
60. Daniel J. Card, "Off-Target Impacts."
61. Jacob Metcalf et al., "AlgorithmicImpact Assessments and Accountability: The Co-construction of Impacts, in Proceedings of the 2021 ACM Conference on Fairness,

Accountability, and Transparency (2021), 735–746; Andrew D. Selbst, "Disparate Impact in Big Data Policing," Georgia Law Review *52* (2017): 109.

62. European Commission, "On Artificial," 25.
63. WHO, *Ethics and Governance*, 66.
64. Leslie et al., *Artificial Intelligence*, 42.
65. Jay Shaw, 2021, *Research Ethics Considerations for the Use of Artificial Intelligence (AI) and Machine Learning (ML) in Health Research*, YouTube video, The Vector Institute, https://youtu.be/nZF0WiikR0w.
66. Card, "Off-Target Impacts."
67. Ibid., 94–95.
68. Ibid., 93.
69. FDA, "About the Patient Representative Program," May 3, 2018, https://www.fda. gov/patients/learn-about-fda-patient-engagement/about-fda-patient-representat ive-program.
70. S. Scott Graham et al., "Assessing Perspectivalism in Patient Participation: An Evaluation of FDA Patient and Consumer Representative Programs," Rhetoric of Health & Medicine *1*, no. 1 (2018): 58–89; 80.
71. Ibid., 79–80.
72. Christa B. Teston et al., "Public Voices in Pharmaceutical Deliberations: Negotiating 'Clinical Benefit' in the FDA's Avastin Hearing," Journal of Medical Humanities *35*, no. 2 (2014): 149–170; Judy Z. Segal, "The Rhetoric of Female Sexual Dysfunction: Faux Feminism and the FDA," Canadian Medical Association Journal *187*, no. 12 (2015): 915–916.
73. Michel Callon, Pierre Lascoumes, and Yannick Barthe, Acting in an Uncertain World: An Essay on Technical Democracy (Cambridge, MA: The MIT Press, 2011), 18.
74. Ibid., 83.
75. McCraddon et al., "Clinical Research," 1326.
76. Xiaoxuan Liu et al., "Reporting Guidelines for Clinical Trial Reports for Interventions Involving Artificial Intelligence: The CONSORT-AI Extension," bmj 370 (2020): m3164.
77. Beau Norgeot et al., "Minimum Information about Clinical Artificial Intelligence Modeling: The MI-CLAIM Checklist," Nature Medicine *26*, no. 9 (2020): 1320–1324.
78. Ibid., 1323.

CHAPTER 8

1. Lynch, *The Origins*.
2. United States National Commission for the Protection of Human Subjects of Biomedical, and Behavioral Research, The Belmont Report: Ethical Principles and Guidelines for the Protection of Human Subjects of Research, Vol. *2* (Washington, DC: The Commission, 1978).
3. It's rare to involve the criminal justice system meaningfully when it comes to pharmaceutical companies, although recent convictions related to the opioid epidemic are one example. Chris Isidore, "OxyContin Maker to Plead Guilty to Federal

Criminal Charges, Pay $8 Billion, and Will Close the Company," *CNN*, October 21, 2020, https://www.cnn.com/2020/10/21/business/purdue-pharma-guilty-plea/index.html.

4. O'Neil, *Weapons*.

5. Benjamin, *Race after*, 81–82; Klein and D'Ignazio, *Data Feminism*, 54–56.

6. Benjamin, *Race after*, 157.

7. Prasad, *Malignant*, 5.

8. Ibid., 34–36.

9. Conant et al., "Improving Accuracy."

10. Han et al., "Deep Neural."

11. Zeevi et al., "Personalized Nutrition."

12. Pierson et al., "Algorithmic Approach."

13. McCraddon et al., "Clinical Research."

14. Liu et al., "Reporting Guidelines;" Norgeot et al., "Minimum Information."

15. Topol, "Welcoming."

16. Hamideh et al., "Your Digital."

17. Norgeot et al., "Minimum Information."

18. Marmot and Wilkinson, *Social Determinants*; WHO Commission on Social Determinants of Health, and World Health Organization, *Closing the Gap*.

19. Hans-Rudolf Berthoud, "The Neurobiology of Food Intake in an Obesogenic Environment," Proceedings of the Nutrition Society *71*, no. 4 (2012): 478–487.

20. Trevor W. Stone, Megan McPherson, and L. Gail Darlington, "Obesity and Cancer: Existing and New Hypotheses for a Causal Connection," EBioMedicine *30* (2018): 14–28.

21. Sacoby Wilson, Malo Hutson, and Mahasin Mujahid, "How Planning and Zoning Contribute to Inequitable Development, Neighborhood Health, and Environmental Injustice," Environmental Justice *1*, no. 4 (2008): 211–216.

22. S. Scott Graham et al., "Catalyzing Transdisciplinarity: A Systems Ethnography of Cancer–Obesity Comorbidity and Risk Coincidence," Qualitative Health Research *27*, no. 6 (2017): 877–892.

23. Jessica Kent, "Addressing the Social Determinants of Health with AI, Partnerships," Health IT Analytics, June 11, 2020, https://healthitanalytics.com/news/addressing-the-social-determinants-of-health-with-ai-partnerships.

24. NIH, "Building Diverse Teams," May 13, 2021, https://commonfund.nih.gov/bridge2ai/enhancingdiverseperspectives#PEDP.

25. London, "Medical Decisions"; Asan et al., "Artificial Intelligence;" Poursabzi-Sangdeh et al., "Manipulating and Measuring."

26. Jay Shaw, "Research Ethics Considerations for the use of Artificial Intelligence (AI) and Machine Learning (ML) in Health Research," 2021, The Vector Institute, YouTube video, https://youtu.be/nZF0WiikR0w.

27. Broussard, *Artificial Unintelligence*.

28. Lynch, *The Origins*, 83.

29. Ibid., 125.

30. Callon et al., *Acting in*.

TECHNICAL APPENDIX

1. Chen et al., "A Support Vector."
2. Max Kuhn et al., "Package 'Caret,'" The R Journal 223 (2020): 7.
3. Liu et al., "A Comparison."
4. Qualitative interpretations are drawn from Mary L. McHugh, "Interrater Reliability: The Kappa Statistic," Biochemia Medica 22, no. 3 (2012): 276–282.
5. Graham and Hopkins, "AI for Social Justice."
6. Kenneth Benoit, Akitaka Matsuo, and Maintainer Kenneth Benoit, "Package 'spacyr'" R package version 0.9 6 (2018).
7. Max Kuhn et al., "Package 'Caret,'" 223.
8. Joses Ho et al., "Moving beyond P Values: Data Analysis with Estimation Graphics," Nature Methods 16, no. 7 (2019): 565–566.
9. Bradley Efron and Robert J. Tibshirani, An Introduction to the Bootstrap (Boca Raton: CRC press, 1994).

Adhiyaman, Vedamurthy, Sonja Adhiyaman, and Radha Sundaram. "The Lazarus Phenomenon." *Journal of the Royal Society of Medicine* 100, no. 12 (2007), 552–557.

AI4People. "On Good AI Governance: 14 Priority Actions, a SMART Model of Governance, and a Regulatory Toolbox." 2019. https://ssrn.com/abstract=3486508.

American Medical Association. "Chapter 8: Opinions on Physicians & The Health of the Community." *AMA Principles of Medical Ethics*. 2001. https://www.ama-assn.org/system/files/2020-12/code-of-medical-ethics-chapter-8.pdf.

American Medical Association. "Organizational Strategic Plan to Embed Racial Justice and Advance Health Equity 2021–2023." 2021. https://www.ama-assn.org/system/files/2021-05/ama-equity-strategic-plan.pdf.

Anand, K.J.S. "Re: Reply to Letters to the Editor from Merskey & Wall." *PAIN* 66, no. 210 (1996), 1438.

Angell, Marcia. *The truth about the Drug companies: How They Deceive Us and What to Do about It*. New York: Random House Incorporated, 2005.

Asan, Onur, Alparslan Emrah Bayrak, and Avishek Choudhury. "Artificial Intelligence and Human Trust in Healthcare: Focus on Clinicians." *Journal of Medical Internet Research* 22, no. 6 (2020), e15154.

Avanti, Anand, Kenneth Jung, Stephanie Harman, Lance Downing, Andrew Ng, and Nigam H. Shah. "Improving Palliative Care with Deep Learning." *arXiv:1711.06402v1* (2017), https://arxiv.org/pdf/1711.06402.pdf.

Aydede, Murat. "Does the IASP Definition of Pain Need Updating?" *PAIN Reports* 4, no. 5 (2019), e777.

Babylon. "AI with 'Imagination' Could Help Doctors with Diagnosis, Particularly for Complex Case." *EurekAlert!* August 11, 2020. https://www.eurekalert.org/pub_releases/2020-08/b-aw081020.php.

Bansal, Gagan, Tongshuang Wu, Joyce Zhu, Raymond Fok, Besmira Nushi, Ece Kamar, Marco Tulio Ribeiro, and Daniel S. Weld. "Does the Whole Exceed Its Parts? The Effect of AI Explanations on Complementary Team Performance." *arXiv:2006.14779* (2020). https://arxiv.org/abs/2006.14779.

Barclay, Andrew Whyte. *A Manual of Medical Diagnosis*. Philadelphia: Blanchard & Lea, 1862.

Becker, Anton S., Michael Mueller, Elina Stoffel, Magda Marcon, Soleen Ghafoor, and Andreas Boss. "Classification of Breast Cancer in Ultrasound Imaging Using a Generic Deep Learning Analysis Software: A Pilot Study." *British Journal of Radiology* 91, no. 1083 (2018), 20170576. https://www.birpublications.org/doi/10.1259/bjr.20170576.

Ben-David, Arie. "About the Relationship between ROC Curves and Cohen's Kappa." *Engineering Applications of Artificial Intelligence* 21, no. 6 (2008), 874–882.

Bender, Emily M., Timnit Gebru, Angelina McMillan-Major, and Margaret Smitchell. "On the Dangers of Stochastic Parrots: Can Language Models Be Too Big?" FAccT, 2021, https://faculty.washington.edu/ebender/papers/Stochastic_Parrots.pdf.

Benjamin, Ruha. "Assessing Risk, Automating Racism." *Science* 366, no. 6464 (2019), 421–422.

Benjamin, Ruha. "Informed Refusal: Toward a Justice-Based Bioethics." *Science, Technology, and Human Values* 43, no. 6 (2016), 967–990.

Benjamin, Ruha. *Race after Technology: Abolitionist Tools for the New Jim Code*. Cambridge: Polity Press, 2019.

Berthoud, Hans-Rudolf. "The Neurobiology of Food Intake in an Obesogenic Environment." *Proceedings of the Nutrition Society* 71, no. 4 (2012), 478–487.

Binghamton University. "Big Data-Driven Method Could Save Money, Increase Efficiency in Pharmaceutical Management." *EurekAlert!* March 29, 2016. https://www.eurekalert.org/pub_releases/2016-03/bu-bdm032916.php.

Blane, Gibert. *A Short Account of the Most Effectual Means of Preserving the Health of Seamen, Particularly in the Royal Navy*. London, 1780.

Bloom, Andrew. "Engineer Bill Baker Is the King of Superstable 150-Story Structures." Wired, November 27, 2007. https://www.wired.com/2007/11/mf-baker/.

Borowsky, Hannah, Leonra Morinis, and Megha Garg. "Disability and Ableism in Medicine: A Curriculum for Medical Students." *MedEd PORTAL* 17, no. 1 (2021), 11073. https://www.mededportal.org/doi/10.15766/mep_2374-8265.11073.

Bower, Joseph L., and Clayton M. Christensen. "Disruptive Technologies: Catching the Wave." *Harvard Business Review*, January–February 1995. https://hbr.org/1995/01/disruptive-technologies-catching-the-wave.

"BPM31510." *Berg Health*. n.d. https://www.berghealth.com/research/healthcare-professionals/pipeline/bpm31510/.

Broussard, Meredith. *Artificial Unintelligence: How Computers Misunderstand the World*. Cambridge, MA: The MIT Press, 2019.

Brown, James M., et al. "Automated Diagnosis of Plus Disease in Retinopathy of Prematurity Using Deep Convolutional Neural Networks." *JAMA Ophthalmology* 136, no. 7 (2018), 803–810, 807.

Buçinca, Zana, Phoebe Lin, Krzysztof Z. Gajos, and Elena L. Glassman. "Proxy Tasks and Subjective Measures Can Be Misleading in Evaluating Explainable AI Systems." In *Proceedings of the 25th International Conference on Intelligent User Interfaces*. pp. 454–464. New York: Association of Computing Machinery, 2020.

Burt, Andrew. "Ethical Frameworks for AI Aren't Enough." *Harvard Business Review*, November 9, 2020. https://hbr.org/2020/11/ethical-frameworks-for-ai-arent-enough.

Callon, Michel, Pierre Lascoumes, and Yannick Barthe. *Acting in an Uncertain World: An Essay on Technical Democracy*. Cambridge, MA: The MIT Press, 2011.

Cani, Patrice D. "Human Gut Microbiome: Hopes, Threats and Promises." *Gut* 67, no. 9 (2018), 1716–1725, 1720.

Caplan, Robyn, Joan Donovan, Lauren Hanson, and Jenna Matthews. *Algorithmic Accountability: A Primer*. Data & Society. 2019. https://datasociety.net/wp-content/uploads/2019/09/DandS_Algorithmic_Accountability.pdf.

Card, Daniel J. "Off-Target Impacts: Tracing Public Participation in Policy Making for Agricultural Biotechnology." *Journal of Business and Technical Communication* 34, no. 1 (2020), 77–103.

Chen, Hui-Ling, Bo Yang, Jie Liu, and Da-You Liu. "A Support Vector Machine Classifier with Rough Set-Based Feature Selection for Breast Cancer Diagnosis." *Expert Systems with Applications* 38, no. 7 (2011), 9014–9022.

Cho, S.I., S. Sun, J.-H. Mun, C. Kim, S.Y. Kim, S. Cho, S.W. Youn, H.C. Kim, and J.H. Chung. "Dermatologist-Level Classification of Malignant Lip Diseases Using a Deep Convolutional Neural Network." *British Journal of Dermatology* 182, no. 6 (2020), 1388–1394.

Cicchetti, Domenic Vincent. "Guidelines, Criteria, and Rules of Thumb for Evaluating Normed and Standardized Assessment Instruments in Psychology." *Psychological Assessment* 6, no. 4 (1994), 284.

Cohen, Jérémie F., Nathalie Bertille, Robert Cohen, and Martin Chalumeau. "Rapid Antigen Detection Tests for Group A Streptococcus in Children with Pharyngitis." *Cochrane Database of Systematic Reviews*, no. 7 (2016), CD010502. doi: 10.1002/14651858.CD010502.pub2.

Compton, Kristin. "Vioxx." *DrugWatch*. n.d. https://www.drugwatch.com/vioxx.

Conant, Emily F., et al. "Association of Digital Breast Tomosynthesis vs Digital Mammography with Cancer Detection and R ecall Rates by Age and Breast Density." *JAMA Oncology* 5, no, 5 (2019), 635–642.

Conant, Emily F., et al. "Improving Accuracy and Efficiency with Concurrent Use of Artificial Intelligence for Digital Breast Tomosynthesis." *Radiology-Artificial Intelligence* 1, no. 4, (2019), e180096.

Cook, Chad, and Charles Sheets. "Clinical Equipoise and Personal Equipoise: Two Necessary Ingredients for Reducing Bias in Manual Therapy Trials." *Journal of Manual & Manipulative Therapy* 19, no. 1 (2011), 55–57.

Corbett-Davies, Sam, and Sharad Goel. "The Measure and Mismeasure of Fairness: A Critical Review of Fair Machine Learning." *arXiv preprint arXiv:1808.00023* (2018). https://arxiv.org/abs/1808.00023.

Daelemans, W. "Part of Speech Tagging." In *Encyclopedia of Machine Learning and Data Mining*. Edited by C. Sammut & G.I., pp. 959. New York: Springer, 2017.

Dafoe, Allan. *AI Governance: A Research Agenda*. Oxford: Centre for the Governance of AI. 2018. https://www.fhi.ox.ac.uk/wp-content/uploads/GovAI-Agenda.pdf.

DeVasto, Danielle. 2016. "Being Expert: L'Aquila and Issues of Inclusion in Science-Policy Decision Making." *Social Epistemology* 30, no. 4, 372–397.

D'Ignazio, Catherine, and Lauren F. Klein. *Data Feminism*. Cambridge, MA: MIT Press, 2020.

Drew, Richard. "IBM Abandons Facial Recognition Products, Condemns Racially Biased Surveillance." NPR. June 9, 2020. https://www.npr.org/2020/06/09/873298 837/ibm-abandons-facial-recognition-products-condemns-racially-biased-surve illance.

Drukker, Karen, Pingkun Yan, Adam Sibley, and Ge Want. "Biomedical Imaging and Analysis through Deep Learning." In *Artificial Intelligence in Medicine*. Edited by Xing, Giger, and Min, 63. 2021.

Efron, Bradley and Robert J. Tibshirani. *An Introduction to the Bootstrap*. Boca Raton: CRC press, 1994.

Eiband, Malin, Daniel Buschek, Alexander Kremer, and Heinrich Hussmann. "The Impact of Placebic Explanations on Trust in Intelligent Systems." In *Extended Abstracts of the 2019 CHI Conference on Human Factors in Computing Systems*. pp. 1–6. New York: Association for Computing Machinery, 2019.

eLife. "New AI Tool Speeds Up Biology and Removes Potential Human Bias." *EurekAlert!* November 2020, https://www.eurekalert.org/pub_releases/2020-11/e-nat110320.php.

Elliott, Carl. *White Coat, Black Hat: Adventures on the Dark Side of Medicine*. Boston: Beacon Press, 2010.

European Commission. "On Artificial Intelligence—a European Approach to Excellence and trust." 2018. https://ec.europa.eu/info/publications/white-paper-artificial-intel ligence-european-approach-excellence-and-trust_en.

Fabi, Rachel, and Daniel S. Goldberg. "Bioethics, (Funding) Priorities, and the Perpetuation of Injustice." *The American Journal of Bioethics* 22, no. 1 (2021), 6–13. https://doi.org/10.1080/15265161.2020.1867934.

Fitzsimons, Gavan J., and Donald R. Lehmann. "Reactance to Recommendations: When Unsolicited Advice Yields Contrary Responses." *Marketing Science* 23, no.1 (2004), 82–94.

Fleiss, Joseph L. *Design and Analysis of Clinical Experiments*. New York: John Wiley & Sons, 2011.

Fleming, Nic. "How Artificial Intelligence Is Changing Drug Discovery." *Nature* 557 (2018), s55–s57.

Food and Drug Administration. "About the Patient Representative Program." 2018. https://www.fda.gov/patients/learn-about-fda-patient-engagement/about-fda-pati ent-representative-program.

Food and Drug Administration. "FDA to iCAD Inc." December 6, 2018. https://www. accessdata.fda.gov/cdrh_docs/pdf18/K182373.pdf.

Food and Drug Administration. "510(k) Clearances." September 2018. https://www.fda. gov/medical-devices/device-approvals-denials-and-clearances/510k-clearances.

Food and Drug Administration. *Guidance for Industry and FDA Staff: Statistical Guidance on Reporting Results from Studies Evaluating Diagnostic Tests*. March 2007. https://www.fda.gov/media/71147/download.

Food and Drug Administration. "Non-Inferiority Clinical Trials to Establish Effectiveness: Guidance for Industry." November 2016. https://www.fda.gov/media/ 78504/download.

Food and Drug Administration. "Proposed Regulatory Framework for Modifications to Artificial Intelligence/Machine Learning (AI/ML)-Based Software as a Medical Device (SaMD): Discussion Paper and Request for Feedback." Accessed April 9, 2021.

https://www.fda.gov/files/medical%20devices/published/US-FDA-Artificial-Intel ligence-and-Machine-Learning-Discussion-Paper.pdf.

FOSTER. "What Is Open Science? Introduction." n.d. https://www.fosteropenscience. eu/content/what-open-science-introduction.

Freedman, David H. "Hunting for New Drugs with AI." *Nature* 576 (2019), s50–s53.

Gabriel, Joseph M. *Medical Monopoly: Intellectual Property Rights and the Origin of the Modern Pharmaceutical Industry.* Chicago: University of Chicago Press, 2014.

Garcia, Denise. "Lethal Artificial Intelligence and Change: The Future of International Peace and Security." *International Studies Review* 20, no. 2 (2018), 334–341.

Gennatas, Efstahios D., and Jonathan H. Chen. "Artificial Intelligence in Medicine: Past, Present, and Future." In *Artificial Intelligence in Medicine: Technical Basis and Clinical Applications.* ed. Xing, Giger, and Min, pp. 3–34, 2021.

Gershgorn, Dave. "Facebook Says It Has a Tool to Detect Bias in Its Artificial Intelligence." *Quartz.* May 3, 2018. https://qz.com/1268520/facebook-says-it-has-a-tool-to-detect-bias-in-its-artificial-intelligence/.

Ghassemi, Marzyeh, Mahima Pushkarna, James Wexler, Jesse Johnson, and Paul Varghese. "Clinicalvis: Supporting Clinical Task-Focused Design Evaluation." *arXiv preprint arXiv:1810.05798* (2018). https://arxiv.org/abs/1810.05798.

Goldberg, Daniel S. "Social Justice, Health Inequalities and Methodological Individualism in US Health Promotion." *Public Health Ethics* 5, no. 2 (2012), 104–115.

Gómez-Valverde, Juan J., et al. "Automatic Glaucoma Classification Using Color Fundus Images Based on Convolutional Neural Networks and Transfer Learning." *Biomedical Optics Express* 10, no. 2 (2019), 892–913.

Google. "ML Fairness Gym." Accessed April 8, 2021.https://github.com/google/ml-fairn ess-gym.

Google. *Perspectives on Issues in AI Governance.* Accessed April 9, 2021. https://ai.goo gle/static/documents/perspectives-on-issues-in-ai-governance.pdf, 2.

Grady, Denise. "A.I. Took a Test to Detect Lung Cancer. It got an A." *The New York Times,* May 20, 2019. https://www.nytimes.com/2019/05/20/health/cancer-artificial-intelligence-ct-scans.html.

Graham, S. Scott. *The Politics of Pain Medicine: A Rhetorical-Ontological Inquiry.* Chicago: University of Chicago Press, 2015.

Graham, S. Scott, Amy Harley, Molly M. Kessler, Laura Roberts, Dannielle DeVasto, Daniel J. Card, Joan M. Neuner, and Sang-Yeon Kim. "Catalyzing Transdisciplinarity: A Systems Ethnography of Cancer–Obesity Comorbidity and Risk Coincidence." *Qualitative Health Research* 27, no. 6 (2017), 877–892.

Graham, S. Scott, and Hannah R. Hopkins. "AI for Social Justice: New Methodological Horizons in Technical Communication." *Technical Communication Quarterly* 31, no. 1 (2021), 89–102.

Graham, S. Scott, Molly M. Kessler, Sang-Yeon Kim, Seokhoon Ahn, and Daniel Card. "Assessing Perspectivalism in Patient Participation: An Evaluation of FDA Patient and Consumer Representative Programs." *Rhetoric of Health & Medicine* 1, no. 1 (2018), 58–89; 80.

Gruss, Sascha, et al. "Pain Intensity Recognition Rates via Biopotential Feature Patterns with Support Vector Machines." *Plos One* (2015), https://doi.org/10.1371/journal.pone.0140330.

Gunn, Lachlan J., François Chapeau-Blondeau, Mark D. McDonnell, Bruce R. Davis, Andrew Allison, and Derek Abbot. "Too Good to be True: When Overwhelming Evidence Fails to Convince." *Proceedings of the Royal Society A* 472, no. 2187 (2016), 20150748. https://doi.org/10.1098/rspa.2015.0748.

Hamideh, Dina, Bianca Arellano, Eric J. Topol, and Steven R. Steinhubl. "Your Digital Nutritionist." *The Lancet* 393, no. 10166 (2019), 19.

Hamilton, Isobel Asher. "Microsoft Took an Ethical Stand on Facial Recognition Just Days after Being Blasted for a Sinister AI Project in China." *Business Insider.* April 17, 2019. https://www.businessinsider.com/microsoft-refuses-to-sell-facial-recognition-tech-to-us-police-force-2019-4.

Han, Seung Seog, Gyeong Hun Park, Woohyung Lim, Myoung Shin Kim, Jung Im Na, Ilwoo Park, and Sung Eun Chang. "Deep Neural Networks Show an Equivalent and Often Superior Performance to Dermatologists in Onychomycosis Diagnosis: Automatic Construction of Onychomycosis Datasets by Region-Based Convolutional Deep Neural Network." *Plos-One* 13, no. 1 (2018), e0191493.

Hao, Karen. "AI Could Make Health Care Fairer—by Helping Us Believe What Patients Say." *MIT Technology Review*, January 22, 2021. https://www.technologyreview.com/2021/01/22/1016577/ai-fairer-healthcare-patient-outcomes/.

Haraway, Donna J. *Modest Witness@Second_Millenium.FemaleMan©_Meets_On coMouse™: Feminism and Technoscience.* New York and London: Routledge, 1997.

Heilman, J.M., Kemmann, E., Bonert, M., Chatterjee, A., Ragar, B., Beards, G.M., Iberri, D.J., et al. 2011. "Wikipedia: A Key Tool for Global Public Health Promotion." *Journal of Medical Internet Research* 13, no. 1, e14.

Hendrickson, Zachary. "Google's DeepMind AI Outperforms Doctors in Identifying Breast Cancer from X-Ray Images." *Business Insider*, January 3, 2020. https://www.businessinsider.com/google-deepmind-outperforms-doctors-identifying-breast-cancer-2020-1.

Herr, Keela, Patrick J Coyne, Tonya Key, Renee Manworren, Margo McCaffery, Sandra Merkel, Jane Pelosi-Kelly, Lori Wild, and American Society for Pain Management Nursing, "Pain Assessment in the Nonverbal Patient: Position Statement with Clinical Practice Recommendations." *Pain Management Nursing* 7, no. 2 (2006), 44–52.

Hilgartner, Stephen. "The Dominant View of Popularization: Conceptual Problems, Political Uses." *Social Studies of Science* 20, no. 3 (1990), 519–539, 519.

Hippocrates. "The Book of Prognostics." Internet Classics Archive. Accessed April 21, 2021. http://classics.mit.edu/Hippocrates/prognost.mb.txt.

Hoffman, Kelly M., Sophie Trawlater, Jordan R. Axt, and M. Norman Oliver. "Racial Bias in Pain Assessment and Treatment Recommendations, and False Beliefs about Biological Differences between Blacks and Whites." *PNAS* 113, no. 16 (2016), 4296–4301.

Howard, Ayanna, Jason Borenstein, and Kinnis Gosha. *NSF-Funded Fairness, Ethics, Accountability, and Transparency (FEAT) Workshop Report.* 2019. https://par.nsf.gov/servlets/purl/10139705.

IBM. *AI Fairness 360*. Accessed April 8, 2021. https://aif360.mybluemix.net.

iCAD. "Artificial Intelligence for Digital Breast Tomosynthesis - Reader Study Results." Revision A. Whitepaper. 2018. https://www.icadmed.com/assets/dmm253-reader-studies-results-rev-a.pdf.

iCAD. "Artificial Intelligence for Digital Breast Tomosynthesis - Reader Study Results." Revision B. Whitepaper. (2020). https://www.icadmed.com/assets/dmm253-reader-studies-results-rev-b.pdf.

iCAD. "iCAD Announces FDA Clearance of ProFound AI™ for Digital Breast Tomosynthesis." December 7, 2018. https://www.icadmed.com/newsroom.html#!/posts/iCAD-Announces-FDA-Clearance-of-ProFound-AI-for-Digital-Breast-Tomosynthesis/124.

iCAD. "iCAD Reports over 1,000 Licenses Sold as Part of ProFound AI Sales." November 24, 2020. https://www.icadmed.com/newsroom.html#!/posts/iCAD-Reports-Over-1000-Licenses-Sold-as-Part-of-ProFound-AI-Sales/232.

iCAD. "ProFound AI® for Digital Breast Tomosynthesis."n.d. https://www.icadmed.com/profoundai.html.

iCAD. "ProFound AI™ for Digital Breast Tomosynthesis."n.d. https://www.icadmed.com/assets/dmm252_profound_ai_for_breast_tomosynthesis_revb.pdf.

iCAD, Inc. "ProFound AI™ for 2D Mammography and Tomosynthesis."n.d. https://pdf.medicalexpo.com/pdf/icad/profound-ai-2d-mammography-tomosynthesis/100519-212559.html.

iCAD. "iCAD Unveils ProFound AI™ for Digital Breast Tomosynthesis at RSNA 2018." November 26, 2018. https://www.icadmed.com/newsroom.html#!/posts/iCAD-Unveils-ProFound-AI-for-Digital-Breast-Tomosynthesis-at-RSNA-2018/123.

ICE Magazine. "iCAD Reports Over 1,000 Licenses Sold as Part of ProFound AI Sales." November 24, 2020, https://theicecommunity.com/icad-reports-over-1000-licenses-sold-as-part-of-profound-ai-sales/.

Institute of Medicine (US) Committee for the Study of the Future of Public Health. *The Future of Public Health*. Washington, DC: National Academies Press (US), 1988. https://www.ncbi.nlm.nih.gov/books/NBK218224.

Ishikawa, Seiji, et al. "Increased Expression of Phosphatidylcholine (16:0/18:1) and (16:0/18:2) in Thyroid Papillary Cancer." *Plos One* (2012). https://doi.org/10.1371/journal.pone.0048873.

Isidore, Chris. "OxyContin Maker to Plead Guilty to Federal Criminal Charges, Pay $8 Billion, and Will Close the Company." CNN, October 21, 2020. https://www.cnn.com/2020/10/21/business/purdue-pharma-guilty-plea/index.html.

Jacobson, Judith S., Victor R. Grann, Dawn Hershman, Andrea B. Troxel, Huling Li, and Alfred I. Neugut. "Breast Biopsy and Race/Ethnicity among Women without Breast Cancer." *Cancer Detection and Prevention* 30, no. 2 (2006), 129–133.

Jaeho Cho, Peter, et al. "Roles of Artificial Intelligence in Wellness, Healthy Living, and Healthy Status Sensing. In *Artificial Intelligence in Medicine*, ed. Xing, Giger, and Min, 151. 2021.

Janz, Heidi L. "Ablesism: The Undiagnosed Malady Afflicting Medicine." *Canadian Association Medical Journal* 191, no. 17 (2019), e478–e479.

Jensen, Jakob D. "Scientific Uncertainty in News Coverage of Cancer Research: Effects of Hedging on Scientists' and Journalists' Credibility." *Human Communication Research* 34, no. 3 (2008), 347–369.

Jillson, Elisa. "Aiming for Truth, Fairness, and Equity in Your Company's Use of AI." FTC. April 19, 2021. https://www.ftc.gov/news-events/blogs/business-blog/2021/04/aiming-truth-fairness-equity-your-companys-use-ai.

Kamath, Preetha, Niteesh Sundaram, Carols Morillo-Hernandez, Fawzy Barry, and Alaina James. "Visual Racism in Internet Searches and Dermatology Textbooks." *Journal of the American Academy of Dermatology*, 85, no. 5 (October 2020), 1348–1349. https://www.sciencedirect.com/science/article/pii/S0190962220328930.

Kaur, Harmmet. "Family of Woman Who Died Weeks after she was Found Alive at a Funeral Home Sues Paramedics for $50 Million." *CNN Online*, October 20, 2020. https://www.cnn.com/2020/10/20/us/timesha-beauchamp-dies-lawsuit-trnd/index.html.

Kellgren, J.H., and J.S. Lawrence. "Radiological Assessment of Osteo-Arthrosis." *Annals of the Rheumatic Diseases* 16 (1957), 494–502. doi: 10.1136/ard.16.4.494.

Kent, Jessica. "Addressing the Social Determinants of Health with AI, Partnerships." *Health IT Analytics*. June 11, 2020. https://healthitanalytics.com/news/addressing-the-social-determinants-of-health-with-ai-partnerships.

Koo, Terry K., and Mae Y. Li. "A Guideline of Selecting and Reporting Intraclass Correlation Coefficients for Reliability Research." *Journal of Chiropractic Medicine* 15, no. 2 (2016), 155–163.

Kuhn, Max, Jed Wing, Steve Weston, Andre Williams, Chris Keefer, Allan Engelhardt, Tony Cooper, Zachary Mayer, Brenton Kenkel, and R. Core Team. "Package 'caret'." *The R Journal* 223 (2020), 7.

Latour, Bruno. *Pandora's Hope: Essays on the Reality of Science Studies*. Cambridge, MA: Harvard University Press, 1999.

Latour, Bruno. *Science in Action: How to Follow Scientists and Engineers through Society*. Cambridge, MA: Harvard University Press, 1987.

Laurance, Jeremy. "The Doctors Had Given Up. They Said Her Heart Had Stopped and She Had Brain Damage. But She's Fine." *The Independent*, October 15, 2012. https://www.independent.co.uk/life-style/health-and-families/health-news/doctors-had-given-they-said-her-heart-had-stopped-and-she-had-brain-damage-she-s-fine-8211015.html.

Lawrence, Halcyon. "Siri Disciplines." In *Your Computer Is on Fire*. Ed. Thomas Mullaney, Benjamin Peters, Mar Hicks, and Kavita Philip, pp. 179–198. Cambridge, MA: The MIT Press, 2021.

"Leading Causes of Death." Centers for Disease Control and Prevention. Last modified January 12, 2021. https://www.cdc.gov/nchs/fastats/leading-causes-of-death.htm.

Lee, Hyunkwant, et al., "An Explainable Deep-Learning Algorithm for the Detection of Acute Intracranial Haemorrhage from Small Datasets." *Nature Biomedical Engineering* 3, no. 3 (2019), 173–182.

Leslie, D., Burr, C., Aitken, M., Cowls, J., Katell, M., and Briggs, M. 2021. *Artificial Intelligence, Human Rights, Democracy, and the Rule of Law: A Primer*. The Council of Europe. https://rm.coe.int/primer-en-new-cover-pages-coe-english-compressed-2754-7186-0228-v-1/1680a2fd4a.

Li, Yingya, Jieke Zhang, and Bei Yu. "An NLP Analysis of Exaggerated Claims in Science News." In *Proceedings of the 2017 EMNLP Workshop: Natural Language Processing Meets Journalism,* pp. 106–111. Copenhagen: Association for Computational Linguistics, Copenhagen, 2017.

"Limitations of Mammograms." American Cancer Society. Last modified October 3, 2019. https://www.cancer.org/cancer/breast-cancer/screening-tests-and-early-detection/mammograms/limitations-of-mammograms.html.

Lin, Rebecca Y., and Jeffery B. Alvarez. "Industry Perspectives and Commercial Opportunities of Artificial Intelligence in Medicine." In *Artificial Intelligence in Medicine.* Ed. Xing, Giger, and Min, 492. 2021.

Lind, James. *An Essay on the Most Effectual Means of Preserving the Health of Seamen, in the Royal Navy.* London: A. Millar, 1757.

Lind, James. *A Treatise on Scurvy in Three Parts.* Edinburgh: Sands, Murray and Conchran, 1753.

Liu, Xiaoxuan, Livia Faes, Aditya U. Kale, Siegfried K. Wagner, Dun Jack Fu, Alice Bruynseels, Thushika Mahendiran, et al. "A Comparison of Deep Learning Performance against Health-Care Professionals in Detecting Diseases from Medical Imaging: A Systematic Review and Meta-Analysis." *The Lancet Digital Health* 1, no. 6 (2019), e271–e297.

Liu, Xiaoxuan, Samantha Cruz Rivera, David Moher, Melanie J. Calvert, and Alastair K. Denniston. "Reporting Guidelines for Clinical Trial Reports for Interventions Involving Artificial Intelligence: The CONSORT-AI Extension." *bmj* 370 (2020), m3164. https://doi.org/10.1136/bmj.m3164.

Lomangino, Kevin. "It's Time for AAAS and EurekAlert! to Crack Down on Misinformation in PR News ReLeases." *Health News Review.* October 2018. https://www.healthnewsreview.org/2018/10/its-time-for-aaas-and-eurekalert-to-crack-down-on-misinformation-in-pr-news-releases/.

London, Alex John. "Medical Decisions: Accuracy versus Explainability." *Hastings Center Report* 49, no. 1, (2019), 15–21.

Long, Erping, et al. "An Artificial Intelligence Platform for the Multihospital Collaborative Management of Congenital Cataracts." *Nature Biomedical Engineering* 1 (2017), 0024.

Longoni, Chiara, and Carey K. Morewedge. AI Can Outperform Doctors. So Why Don't Patients Trust it? *Harvard Business Review,* October 30, 2019. https://hbr.org/2019/10/ai-can-outperform-doctors-so-why-dont-patients-trust-it.

Lyell, David, Enrico Coiera, Jessica Chen, Parina Shah, and Farah Magrabi. "How Machine Learning Is Embedded to Support Clinician Decision Making: An Analysis of FDA-Approved Medical Devices." *BMJ Health & Care Informatics* 28, no. 1 (2021), e100301. doi: 10.1136/bmjhci-2020-100301..

Lynch, John A. *The Origins of Bioethics: Remembering When Medicine Went Wrong.* East Lansing: MSU Press, 2019.

Lynch, John, Desiré Bennett, Alison Luntz, Courtney Toy, and Eva VanBenschoten. "Bridging Science and Journalism: Identifying the Role of Public Relations in the

Construction and Circulation of Stem Cell Research among Laypeople." *Science Communication* 36, no. 4 (2014), 479–501.

Mandrekar, Jayawant N. "Receiver Operating Characteristic Curve in Diagnostic Test Assessment." *Journal of Thoracic Oncology* 5, no. 9 (2010), 1315–1316.

Marmot, Michael, and Richard Wilkinson, eds. *Social Determinants of Health.* Oxford: OUP, 2005.

Master, Farah. "Computing Industry CO2 Emissions in the Spotlight." *Reuters.* January 15, 2009. https://www.reuters.com/article/us-computing-carbon-emissions/comput ing-industry-co2-emissions-in-the-spotlight-idUSTRE50E5QO20090115.

Matheny, M., S. Thadaney Israni, and M. Ahmed. *Artificial Intelligence in Health Care: The Hope, the Hype, the Promise, the Peril.* Washington, DC: National Academy of Medicine, 2019.

McCradden, Melissa D., Shalmali Joshi, Mjaye Mazawi, and James A. Anderson. "Ethical Limitations of Algorithmic Fairness Solutions in Health Care Machine Learning." *The Lancet Digital Health* 2, no. 5 (2020), E221–E223.

McCradden, Melissa D., Elizabeth A. Stephenson, and James A. Anderson. "Clinical Research Underlies Ethical Integration of Healthcare Artificial Intelligence." *Nature Medicine* 26, no. 9 (2020), 1325–1326.

McHugh, Mary L. "Interrater Reliability: The Kapp Statistic." *Biochemia Medica* 22, no. 3, (2012), 276–282.

McKinney, Scott Mayer, et al. "International Evaluation of an AI System for Breast Cancer Screening." *Nature* 577 (2020), 89–94, 89.

Meskó, Berci. Twitter post. March 23, 2021, 10:00 a.m. twitter.com/Berci/status/1374375523082629143.

Metz, Cade. "Google Says Its AI Catches 99.9 Percent of Gmail Spam." *Wired,* July 9, 2015. https://www.wired.com/2015/07/google-says-ai-catches-99-9-percent-gmail-spam/.

Micca, Peter, Christine Chang, Simon Gisby, and Maulesh Shulka. "Trends in Health Yech Investments: Funding the Future of Health." *Deloitte Insights.* February 26, 2021. https://www2.deloitte.com/us/en/insights/industry/health-care/health-tech-private-equity-venture-capital.html.

Mini-Mental State Exam (MMSE). Retrieved February 2021. https://www.ncbi.nlm.nih.gov/projects/gap/cgi-bin/GetPdf.cgi?id=phd001525.1.

Mitchell, Alex J. "A Meta-Analysis of the Accuracy of the Mini-Mental State Examination in the Detection of Dementia and Mild Cognitive Impairment." *Journal of Psychiatric Research* 43, no. 4 (2008), 411–431.

Mitchell, Tom, M. "The Discipline of Machine Learning," 2006, http://www.cs.cmu.edu/~tom/pubs/MachineLearning.pdf.

Mullaney, Thomas. "Your Computer Is on Fire." In *Your Computer Is on Fire.* Edited by Thomas Mullaney, Benjamin Peters, Mar Hicks, and Kavita Philip pp. 3–10. Cambridge, MA: The MIT Press, 2021.

Neilson, Shane. "Ableism in the Medical Profession." *Canadian Association Medical Journal* 192, no. 15 (2020), e411–e412.

NIH. "Building Diverse Teams." May 13, 2021. https://commonfund.nih.gov/bridge2ai/enhancingdiverseperspectives#PEDP.

Noble, Safiya Umoja. *Algorithms of Oppression: How Search Engines Reinforce Racism.* New York: New York University Press, 2018.

Norgeot, Beau, Giorgio Quer, Brett K. Beaulieu-Jones, Ali Torkamani, Raquel Dias, Milena Gianfrancesco, Rima Arnaout, et al. "Minimum Information about Clinical Artificial Intelligence Modeling: The MI-CLAIM Checklist." *Nature Medicine* 26, no. 9 (2020), 1320–1324.

Northwestern University. "AI Tools Speeds Up Search for COVID-19 Treatments and Vaccines." *EurekAlert!* May 4, 2020. https://www.eurekalert.org/pub_releases/2020-05/nu-ats042920.php.

O'Dwyer, Laurence, et al. "Using Support Vector Machines with Multiple Indices of Diffusion for Automated Classification of Mild Cognitive Impairment." *PLoS-One* 7, no. 2 (2012), e32441.

O'Hare, Ryan. "Artificial Intelligence Could Help to Spot Breast Cancer." Imperial College London. January 2020. https://www.imperial.ac.uk/news/194506/artificial-intelligence-could-help-spot-breast/.

O'Neil, Cathy. *Weapons of Math Destruction: How Big Data Increases Inequality and Threatens Democracy.* New York: Crown, 2016.

Oransky, Ivan. "NIH Suspended Some Grants to Duke amid Concern for Patient Safety." Medscape. May 21, 2019. https://www.medscape.com/viewarticle/913283.

Panesar, Arjun. Machine Learning and AI for Healthcare: Big Data for Improved Health Outcomes. 2nd ed. Berkeley, CA: Apress, 2021.

Pasquale, Frank. *New Laws of Robotics.* Cambridge, MA: Harvard University Press, 2020.

Patro, Jasabanta, and Sabyasachee Baruah. "A Simple Three-Step Approach for the Automatic Detection of Exaggerated Statements in Health Science News." In *Proceedings of the 16th Conference of the European Chapter of the Association for Computational Linguistics: Main Volume.* pp. 3293–3305. Association for Computational Linguistics, 2021.

Phelps, Jordyn. "Trump Keeps Bragging about Acing Simple Test Used to Detect Mental Impairment." *ABC News*, July 23, 2020. https://abcnews.go.com/Politics/trump-bragging-acing-simple-test-detect-mental-impairment/story?id=71945342.

Philip, Kvita. "How to Stop Worrying about Clean Signals." In *Your Computer Is on Fire.* Edited by Thomas Mullaney, Benjamin Peters, Mar Hicks, and Kavita Philip, 368–369. Cambridge, MA: The MIT Press, 2021.

Pierson, Emma, David M. Cutler, Jure Leskovec, Sendhil Mullainathan, and Ziad Obermeyer. "An Algorithm Approach to Reducing Unexplained Pain Disparities in Underserved Populations." *Nature Medicine* 27 (2021), 136–140.

Pontika, Nancy, Petr Knoth, Matteo Cancellieri, and Samuel Pearce. "Fostering Open Science to Research Using a Taxonomy and an eLearning Portal." Paper presented at iKnow: 15th International Conference on Knowledge Technologies and Data Driven Business, Graz, Austria, October 21–22, 2015.

Poslusny, Catherine. "How Much Does a PET Scan Cost?" *New Choice Health.* Accessed April 8, 2021. https://www.newchoicehealth.com/pet-scan/cost.

Poursabzi-Sangdeh, Forough, Daniel G. Goldstein, Jake M. Hofman, Jennifer Wortman Vaughan, and Hanna Wallach. 2021. "Manipulating and Measuring Model Interpretability." In *CHI Conference on Human Factors in Computing Systems. (CHI*

'21), May 8–13, 2021, Yokohama, Japan. New York: ACM, 2021. https://doi.org/10.1145/3411764.3445315.

Prasad, Vinayak K. *Malignant: How Bad Policy and Bad Evidence Harm People with Cancer.* Baltimore: Johns Hopkins University Press, 2020.

Prasad, Vinayak K., and Adam S. Cifu. *Ending Medical Reversal: Improving Outcomes, Saving Lives.* Baltimore: Johns Hopkins University Press, 2015.

Prasad, Vinay, and Adam Cifu. "Medical Reversal: Why We Must Raise the Bar before Adopting New Technologies." *Yale Journal of Biology and Medicine* 84, no. 4 (2011), 471–478.

Price, Catherine. "The Age of Scurvy." *Distillations* 3, no. 2 (2018), 12–23.

Radiology Society of North America (RSNA). "RSNA 2020 Booth Space Selection Guidelines." n.d. https://www.rsna.org/-/media/Files/RSNA/Annual-meeting/Exhibitors/Tools-and-guides/2020-booth-space-selection-guidelines_final.ashx.

Raja, Srinivasa, et al. "The Revised International Association for the Study of Pain Definition of Pain: Concepts, Challenges, and Compromises." *PAIN* 161, no. 9 (2020), 1976–1982.

Raji, Inioluwa Deborah, Andrew Smart, Rebecca N. White, Margaret Mitchell, Timnit Gebru, Ben Hutchinson, Jamila Smith-Loud, Daniel Theron, and Parker Barnes. "Closing the AI Accountability Gap: Defining an End-to-End Framework for Internal Algorithmic Auditing." In *Proceedings of the 2020 Conference on Fairness, Accountability, and Transparency.* pp. 33–44. New York: Association for Computing Machinery.

Reader, Ruth. "Why Google, Amazon, and Nvidia Are All Building AI Notetakers for Doctors." November 13, 2020. https://www.fastcompany.com/90555218/google-amazon-nvidia-ai-medical-transcription.

Reynolds, Joel Michael. "Three Things Clinicians Should Know about Disability." *AMA Journal of Ethics* 20, no. 12, e1181–e1187.

Rogers, Everett. *Diffusion of Innovations* New York: Free Press, 2003.

Romero-Brufau, Santiago, Kim Gaines, Clara T. Nicolas, Matthew G. Johnson, Joel Hickman, and Jeanne M. Huddleston. "The Fifth Vital Sign? Nurse Worry Predicts Inpatient Deterioration within 24 hours." *JAMIA Open* 2, no. 4 (2019), 465–470.

Rowe, Gene, and Lynn J. Frewer. "A Typology of Public Engagement Mechanisms." *Science, Technology, & Human Values* 30, no. 2 (2005), 251–290.

Sabin, Janice A. "How We Fail Black Patients in Pain." Association of American Medical Colleges. January 6, 2020. https://www.aamc.org/news-insights/how-we-fail-black-patients-pain.

Sayres, Rory, et al. "Using a Deep Learning Algorithm and Integrated Gradients Explanation to Assist Grading for Diabetic Retinopathy." *Ophthalmology* 126, no. 4 (2019), 552–564.

Schmidt-Erfurth, Ursula, Amir Sadeghipour, Bianca S. Gerendas, Sebastian M. Waldstein, and Hrvoje Bogunović. "Artificial Intelligence in Retina." *Progress in Retinal and Eye Research* 67 (2018), 1–29.

Schultz, Myron. "Rudolf Virchow." *Emerging Infectious Diseases* 14, no. 9 (2008), 1480–1481.

Segal, Judy Z. "The Rhetoric of Female Sexual Dysfunction: Faux Feminism and the FDA." *CMAJ* 187, no. 12 (2015), 915–916.

Shapiro, Joseph. "People with Disabilities Fear Pandemic Will Worsen Medical Biases." NPR. April 15, 2020. https://www.npr.org/2020/04/15/828906002/people-with-disab ilities-fear-pandemic-will-worsen-medical-biases.

Shaw, Jay. *Research Ethics Considerations for the Use of Artificial Intelligence (AI) and Machine Learning (ML) in Health Research*. YouTube video. The Vector Institute. 2021. https://youtu.be/nZF0WiikR0w.

Simple Life. "Simple Fasting App Will Provide Personalized Dieting Tips through AI-powered Functionality." *Cision PR Newswire*, February 4, 2020. https://www.prnewsw ire.com/news-releases/simple-fasting-app-will-provide-personalized-dieting-tips-through-ai-powered-functionality-300996820.html.

Smith, Robert J., and Brittany U. Oliver. "Advocating for Black Lives—a Call to Dermatologists to Dismantle Institutionalized Racism and Address Racial Health Inequities." *JAMA Dermatology*, 157, no 2 (November 2020), 155–156. https://jama network.com/journals/jamadermatology/article-abstract/2773122.

Soares, M.J., M.J. Müller, H. Boeing, C. Maffeis, A. Misra, G. Muscogiuri, S. Muthayya, P. Newsholme, T. Wolever, and S. Zhu. "Conflict of Interest in Nutrition Research: An Editorial Perspective." *European Journal of Clinical Nutrition* 73 (2019), 1213–1215.

Stanton, Lisa J., et al. "When Race Matters: Disagreements in Pain Perception between Patients and Their Physicians in Primary Care." *Journal of the National Medical Association* 99, no. 5 (2007), 532–838.

Star Trek: The Next Generation. "The Naked Now." #40271-103. Episode 3. Written by D.C. Fontana and Gene Roddenberry. June 1987.

STAT. "Promise and Peril: How Artificial Intelligence Is Transforming Healthcare." 2021. https://www.statnews.com/wp-content/uploads/2021/04/STAT_Promise_and_Peril_2021_Report.pdf, 13.

Stevens, Adam R.H., Sabine Bellstedt, Pascal J. Elahi, and Michael T. Murphy. "The Imperative to Reduce Carbon Emissions in Astronomy." *Nature Astronomy* 4 (2020), 843–851.

Stone, Trevor W., Megan McPherson, and L. Gail Darlington. "Obesity and Cancer: Existing and New Hypotheses for a Causal Connection." *EBioMedicine* 30 (2018), 14–28.

Teston, Christa B., S. Scott Graham, Raquel Baldwinson, Andria Li, and Jessamyn Swift. "Public Voices in Pharmaceutical Deliberations: Negotiating 'Clinical Benefit' in the FDA's Avastin Hearing." *Journal of Medical Humanities* 35, no. 2 (2014), 149–170.

Thoma, Martin. "Receiver Operating Characteristic (ROC) Curve with False Positive Rate and True Positive Rate." June 24, 2018. https://en.wikipedia.org/wiki/Receiver_o perating_characteristic#/media/File:Roc-draft-xkcd-style.svg.

Thomas, John M., Leo M. Cooney, and Terri R. Fried. "Prognosis Reconsidered in Light of Ancient Insights—from Hippocrates to Modern Medicine." *JAMA Internal Medicine* 179, no. 6 (2019), 820–823, 820.

Topol, Eric. *Deep Medicine: How Artificial Intelligence Can Make Healthcare Human Again*. New York: Basic Books, 2019.

Topol, Eric J. "Welcoming New guidelines for AI Clinical Research." *Nature Medicine* 26, no. 9 (2020), 1318–1320, 1319.

Tutt, Andrew. "An FDA for Algorithms." *Administrative Law Review* 69 (2017), 83.

Underwood, A. "Fibromyalgia: Not all in your head." *Newsweek*, May 19, 2003, 53.

United States National Commission for the Protection of Human Subjects of Biomedical, and Behavioral Research. *The Belmont Report: Ethical Principles and Guidelines for the Protection of Human Subjects of Research*. Vol. 2. The Commission. Washington , DC: US Government Printing Office, 1978.

Velazco, Chris. "Facebook Can't Move Fast to Fix the Things It Broke." *Engadget*. April 12, 2018. https://www.engadget.com/2018-04-12-facebook-has-no-quick-solutions.html.

Walsh, Fergus. "AI 'Outperforms' Doctors Diagnosing Breast Cancer." *BBC News*, January 2, 2020. https://www.bbc.com/news/health-50857759.

WHO. *Ethics and Governance of Artificial Intelligence for Health: WHO Guidance*. Geneva: World Health Organization, 2021.

WHO Commission on Social Determinants of Health, and World Health Organization. *Closing the Gap in a Generation: Health Equity through Action on the Social Determinants of Health: Commission on Social Determinants of Health Final Report*. Geneva: World Health Organization, 2008.

WHO Scientific Group. *Guidelines for Evaluation of Drugs for Use in Man*. Geneva: World Health Organization, 1975.

"William F. Baker (Engineer)." *Wikipedia*. Accessed February 28, 2021. https://en.wikipedia.org/wiki/William_F._Baker_(engineer).

Wilson, Sacoby, Malo Hutson, and Mahasin Mujahid. "How Planning and Zoning Contribute to Inequitable Development, Neighborhood Health, and Environmental Injustice." *Environmental Justice* 1, no. 4 (2008), 211–216.

Wolever, T.M.S. "Personalized Nutrition by Prediction of Glycaemic Responses: Fact or Fantasy?" *European Journal of Clinical Nutrition* 70, no. 4 (2016), 411–413.

Wong, Andrew, Erkin Otles, John P. Donnelly, Andrew Krumm, Jeffrey McCullough, Olivia DeTroyer-Cooley, Justin Pestrue, et al. "External Validation of a Widely Implemented Proprietary Sepsis Prediction Model in Hospitalized Patients." *JAMA Internal Medicine* 181, no. 8 (2021), 1065–1070.

World Health Organization. "Smallpox Vaccines." May 31, 2016. https://www.who.int/news-room/feature-stories/detail/smallpox-vaccines.

Wu, Eric, Kevin Wu, Roxana Daneshjou, David Ouyang, Daniel E. Ho, and James Zou. "How Medical AI Devices Are Evaluated: Limitations and Recommendations from an Analysis of FDA Approvals." *Nature Medicine* 27, (2021), 582–584.

Xing, Lei, Maryellen L. Giger, and James K. Min, eds. *Artificial Intelligence in Medicine: Technical Basis and Clinical Applications*. London: Academic Press, 2021.

Yang, Yin, Yiping Ge, Lifang Guo, Qiuju Wu, Lin Peng, Erjia Zhang, Junxiang Xie, et al. "Development and Validation of Two Artificial Intelligence Models for Diagnosing Benign, Pigmented Facial Skin Lesions." *Skin Research and Technology*, 27, no 1 (August 2020), 74–79. https://doi.org/10.1111/srt.12911.

Yerushalmy, Jacob. "Statistical Problems in Assessing Methods of Medical Diagnosis, with Special Reference to X-Ray Techniques." *Public Health Reports (1896–1970)* 62, no. 40 (1947), 1432–1449.

Yu, Bei, Jun Wang, Lu Guo, and Yingya Li. "Measuring Correlation-to-Causation Exaggeration in Press Releases." In *Proceedings of the 28th International Conference on Computational Linguistics.* Edited by Donia Scott, Nuria Bel, Chengqing Zong. pp. 4860–4872. Barcelona: International Committee on Computational Linguistics, 2020.

Zeevi, David, Tal Korem, Niv Zmora, David Israeli, Daphna Rothschild, Adina Weinberger, Orly Ben-Yacov, et al. "Personalized Nutrition by Prediction of Glycemic Responses." *Cell* 163, no. 5 (2015), 1079–1094.

Zeng, Daniel, Zhidong Cao, and Daniel B. Neill. "Artificial Intelligence—Enabled Public Health Surveillance—from Local Detection to Global Epidemic Monitoring." In *Artificial Intelligence in Medicine: Technical Basis and Clinical Applications.* Edited by Lei Xing, Maryellen L. Giger, and James K. Min. pp. 437–454. London: Academic Press, 2021.

Zhang, Chao, et al. "Toward an Expert Level of Lung Cancer Detection and Classification Using a Deep Convolutional Neural Network." *The Oncologist* 24, no. 9 (2019), 1159–1165.

Zhou, Li, and Margarita Sordo. "Expert Systems in Medicine." In *Artificial Intelligence in Medicine,* 75–100.

Zyga, Lisa. "Why Too Much Evidence Can Be a Bad Thing." *Phys.org.* January 4, 2016. https://phys.org/news/2016-01-evidence-bad.html.

For the benefit of digital users, indexed terms that span two pages (e.g., 52–53) may, on occasion, appear on only one of those pages.

Tables and Figures are indicated by *t* and *f* following the page number

VAS. *See* Visual Analog Scale (VAS)
verbs, modal, 131–32
Verghese, Abraham, 1, 5
Vioxx, 69–70
Virchow, Rudolf, 44
Visual Analog Scale (VAS), 136–37
voice-activated technology, 31–32

war robots, 141
Weapons of Math Description (O'Neil), 10–11, 13–14, 139, 164–65
Weapons of Math Description (WMD), 10, 13–14, 15, 186–92, 188t
White Coat, Black Hat (Elliott), 71–72

Wikipedia, 55–56
Wisconsin Breast Cancer Dataset (WBDC), 31–32, 33, 37–38, 104–5
women, fibromyalgia in, 151, 152
writing, science, 113–14, 119, 131–33. *See also* press releases

XAI. *See* eXplainable AI (XAI)

Yerushalmy, Jacob, 45
Yoon, Sang Won, 116
Your Computer Is on Fire (Mullaney), 140–41, 144
Yunus, Muhammad, 151